LaLa Salama

——— AND ———
OTHER SAVASANA READINGS

COLLEEN ANNE TORIANNE

Poems and illustrations by Colleen Anne Torianne.
Prepared for Publishing by Mindee Thyrring.

Dedication
for the child within

Lala Salama

I fell asleep to the lullaby of the tree frogs.

"Lala salama," they sang
"Lighten the night with
your sweetest of dreams"

So I dreamt I found my
way to the river in
the deepest dark of the
jungle. The stardust I
found in my pocket and
tossed in the air became
a thousand fire flies that
lit the way. They were all
there at the river's edge:
the bears, the big cats, the
rabbit, the deer, even
the cobra.   "It's safe here,"
they said "We don't need to
beat the drums. They just play."
And, on that endless night
we danced by the river;
we didn't miss the sun.

I fell awake to the coda of the morning birds.

"Lala salama" they sang
"Brighten the day with
your sweetest of dreams"

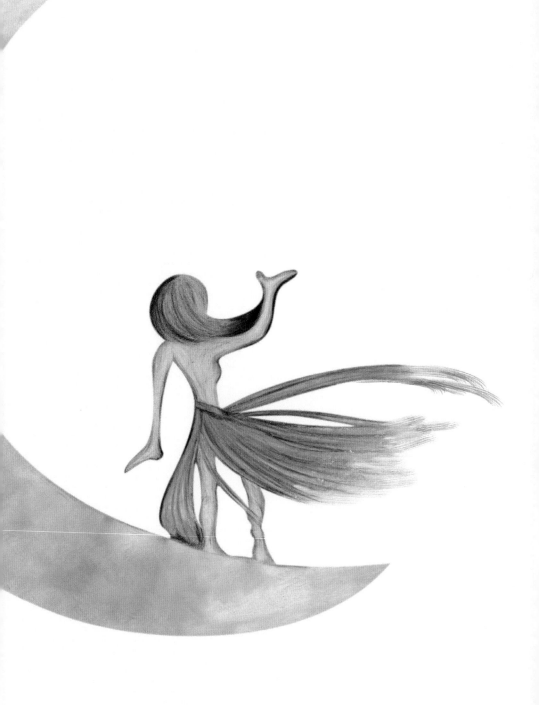

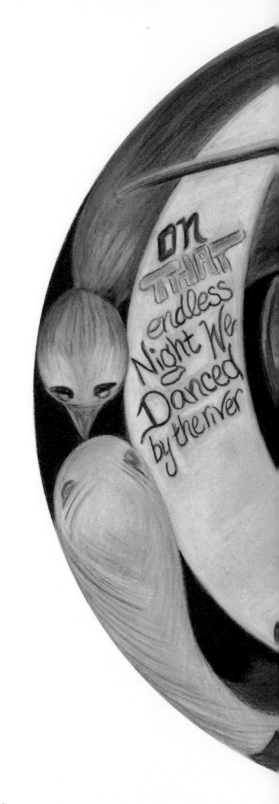

"Lala salama"
they sang!

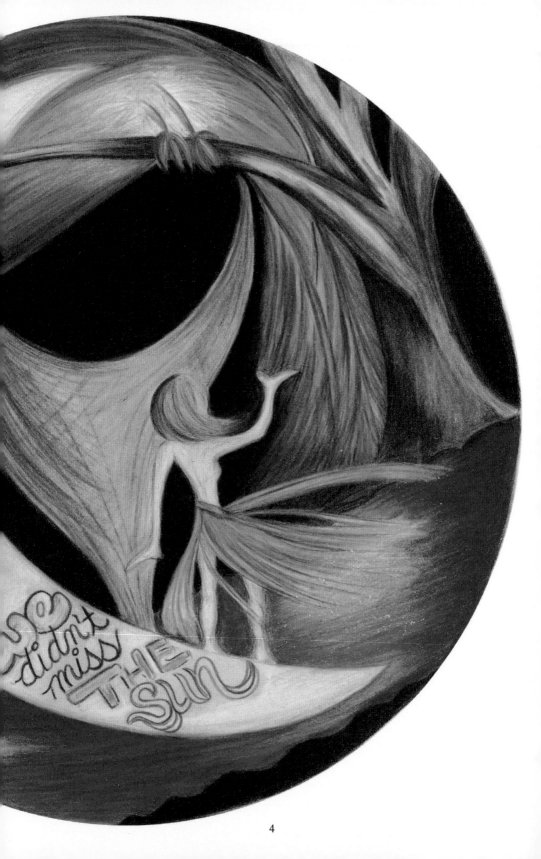

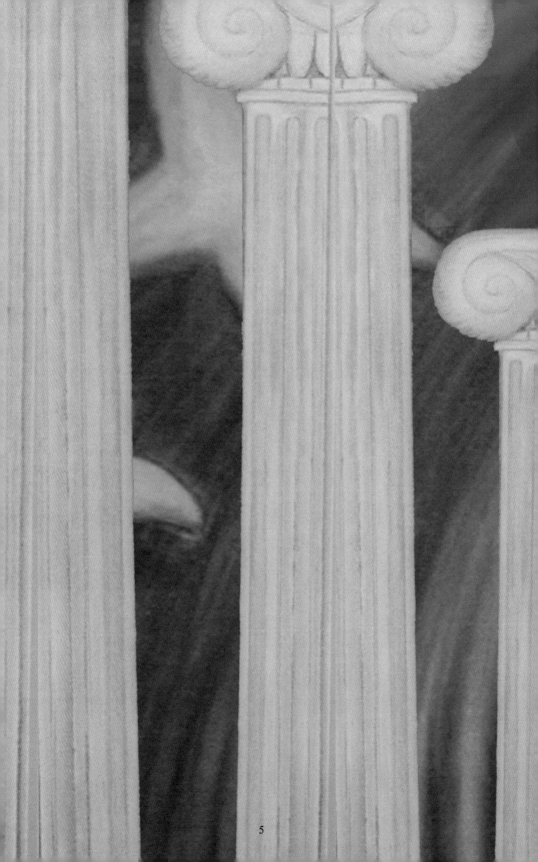

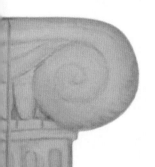

Erasing Time

I lie in the desert where
the wind erased time. Turquoise
air spins my silver toe ring into
gold; my feet turn to sand and
blow away. Once ankles, shins,
knees, thighs, now amber shapes of
these lift grain by grain to twirl,
sparkle, go. Hips unravel
in a cloud, arms sift out through
fingers, drifting to distant
dunes. I inhale. I exhale.
A burst of gold dust scatters
heart and spine and face and mind.
A light dances at the crown
of my head.   It grows smaller,
flickers, goes out.
I am the desert wind erasing time.

*I am
the desert wind
erasing time*

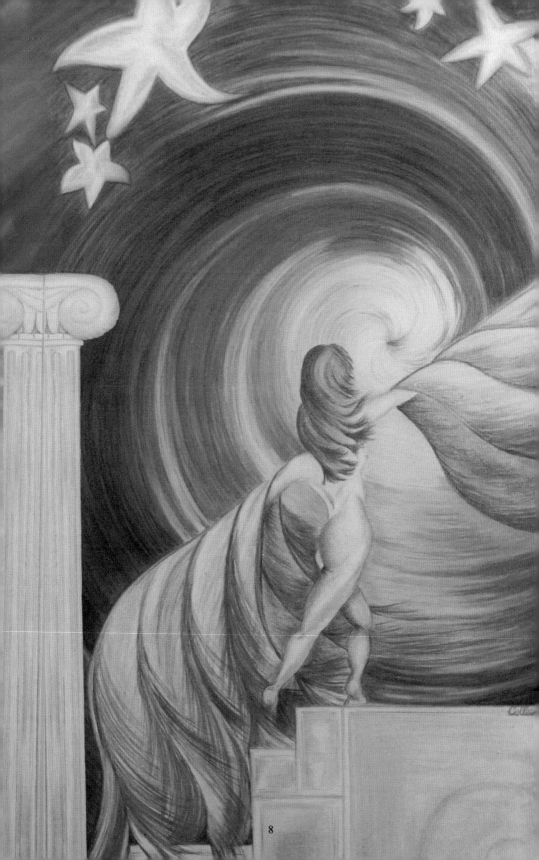

8

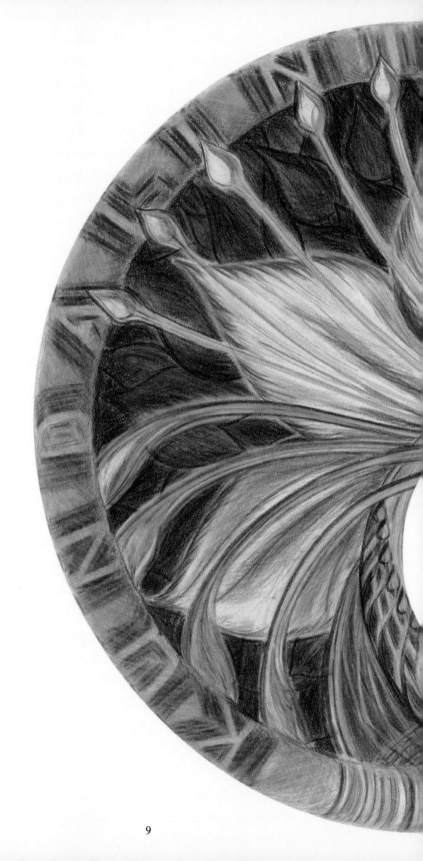

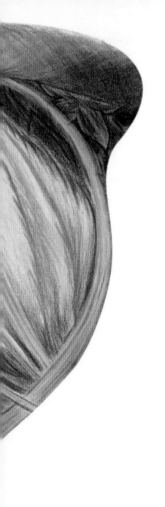

Comet Back to Earth

Every time I make the journey,
I wonder why I ever leave.
I take a magic carpet ride
beyond the sea, beyond the sky,
to those places I almost know
where I can be warm in the snow,
cry with tears that water my soul,
run through sunny puddles of rain,
sleep through the frog cricket chorus,
as we speak of things without words.
I catch a comet back to earth
but don't seem to notice until
the next time I make the journey
and wonder why I ever leave.

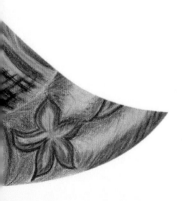

Magic Carpet Ride

Just before dawn, the white owl
appears. We soar past the sun
rise to the sea. A blue whale
takes us beyond pink and green
gardens of coral and eels
to the vast desert on the
other side. A thousand dunes
by camel carry us back
before time to see shooting
stars that become you and I.

We travel far and wide, deep
inside without leaving at
all; not just a yoga mat
but a magic carpet ride.

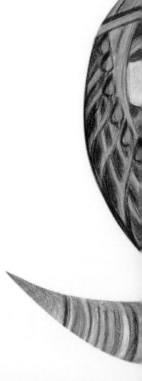

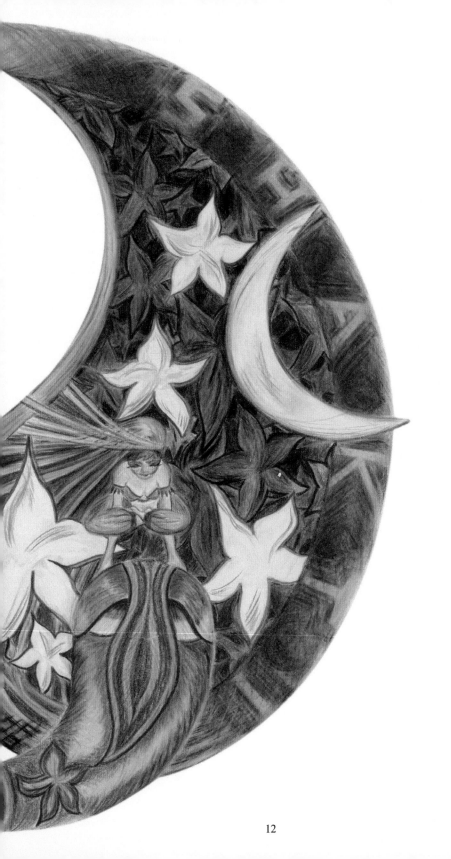

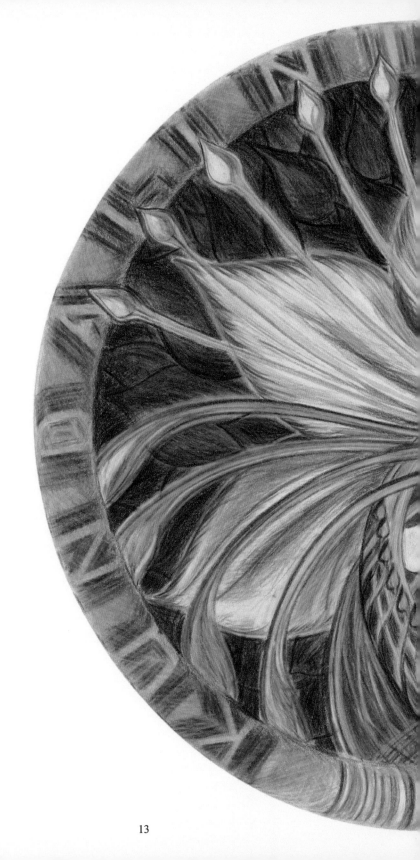

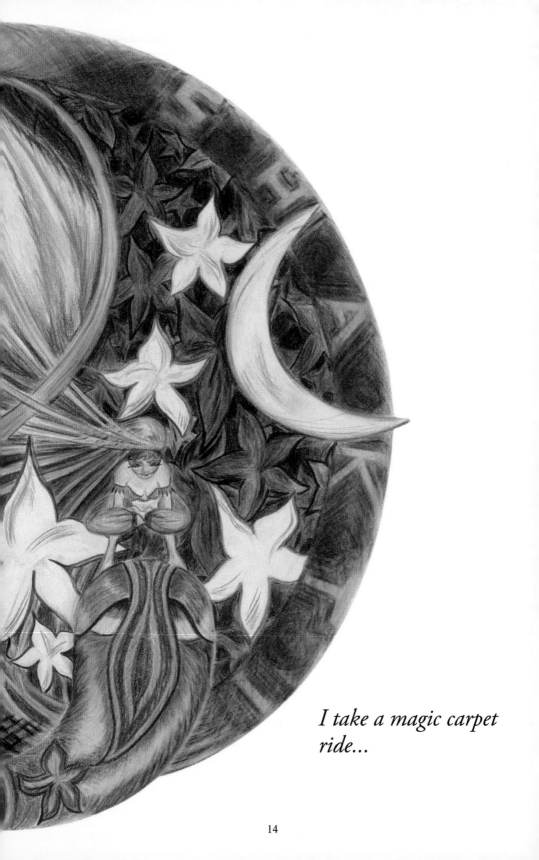

I take a magic carpet ride...

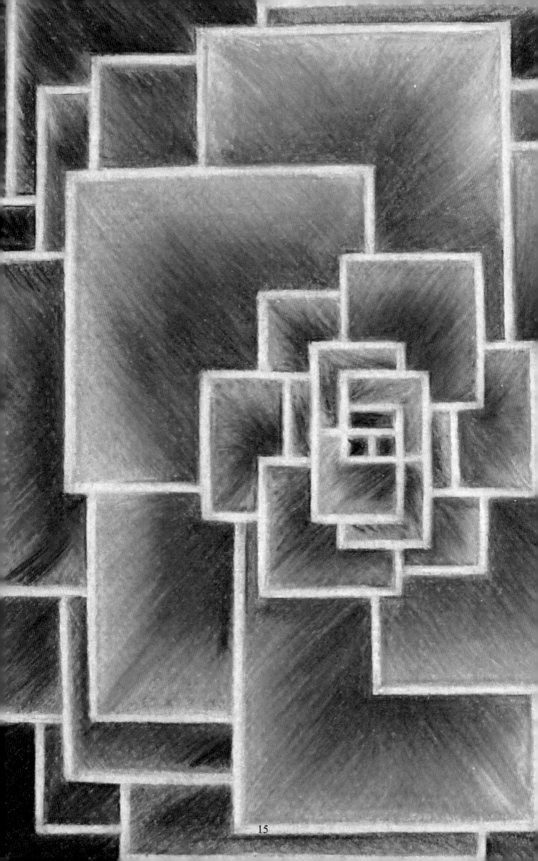

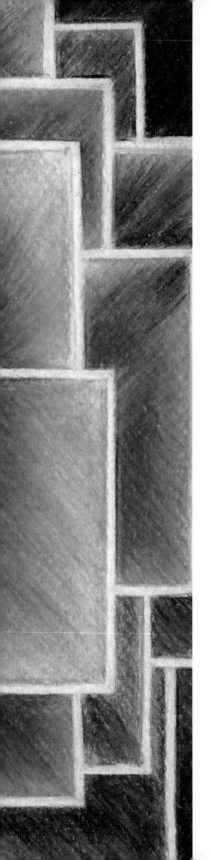

Rainy Days

I follow my heart and it leads me here
across the bluffs in the rain. I
can not see or hear the waves but
I remember how I will find you

Fog blurs the sky and land into one grey,
as wind whispers truth in my ears.
I walk into this misted dream
where time is marked
by your beating heart

I move in circles and lose my way; this
is the way I know to find you.
Just when you seem furthest away
you're by my side
where you'd always be

if I wouldn't forget and let bright sun
get in my eyes.   It takes clouds to
soften the glare and show me where
you wait for me
on those rainy days.

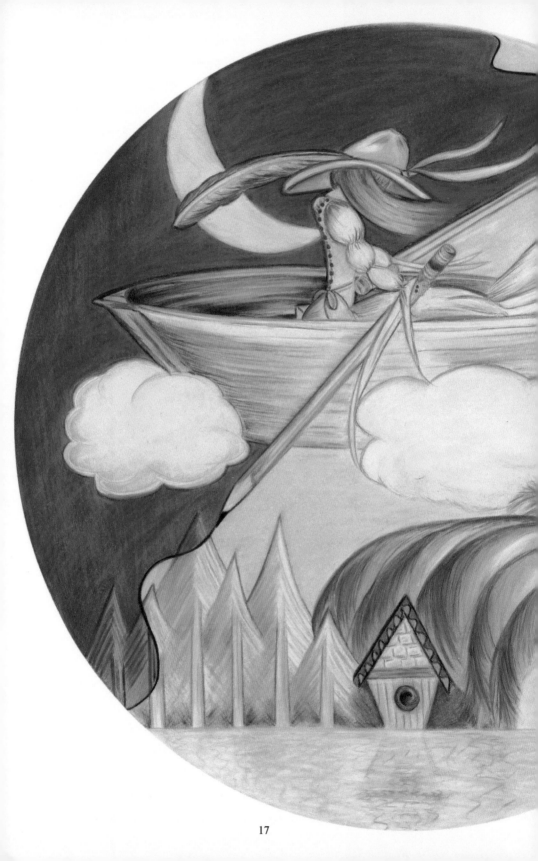

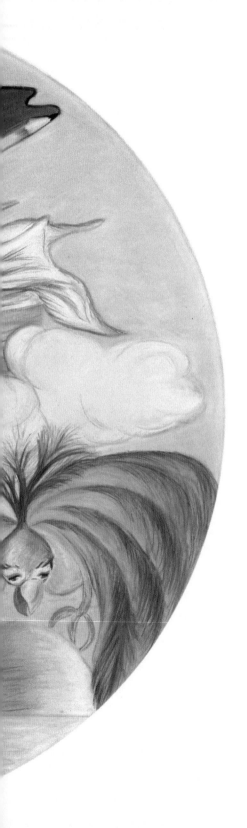

Time Travel

Where does the time go
and where does it come from?

I went early so I
might see myself arrive.
But, when I got there I was
just leaving.   In a boat

I rowed across the sky,
against the wind.   But, when
I missed the sun as it set,
I ran through rain and tears

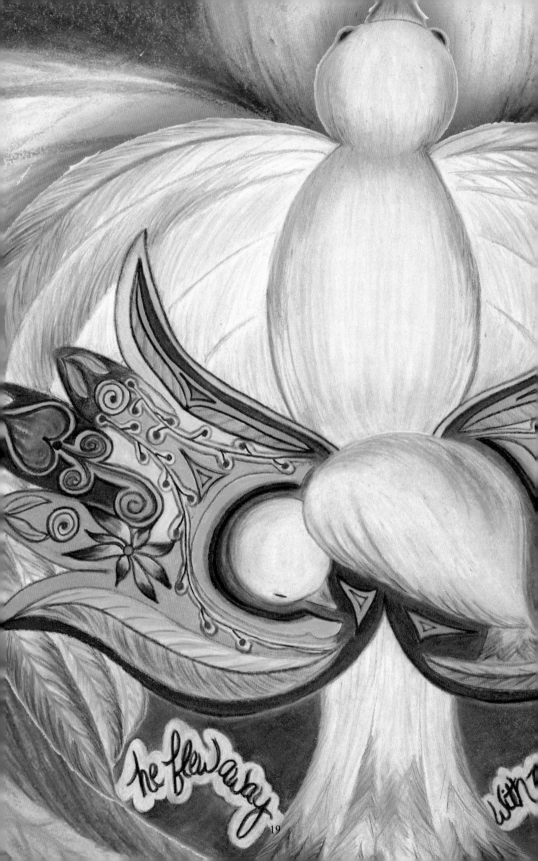

he flew away

with

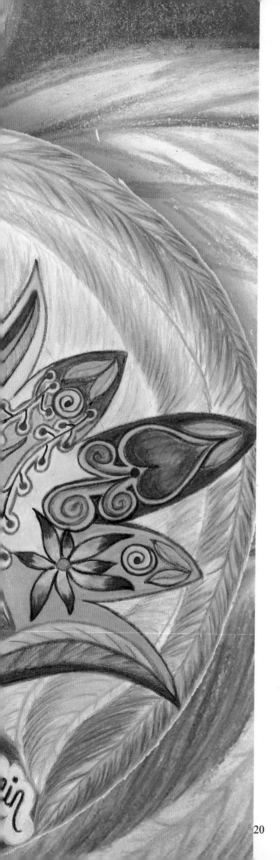

to my door, where I held
the bird that died on the
step. And, when the sun rose, he
flew away with my pain.

Someday they will google
and learn once there wasn't
a Google at all. That's when
they'll make the time to come

back and sit as we tell
stories of grandparents
and those who came before.
Then,
we'll ask the travelers,

"Where does the time go
and where does it come from?"

Moment to Moment

From nowhere there is a moment so free
and I am one with the air and the sea.
The moment is gone.
But,
lost in a worry,
fast with hurry,
the traffic queue,
the endless list to do
are merely moments too

By chance and by grace here's another like this:
as if time is locked in the lover's kiss.
The moment is gone.
But,

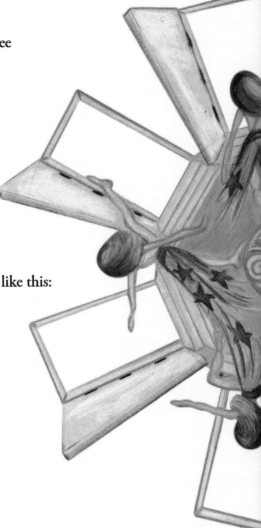

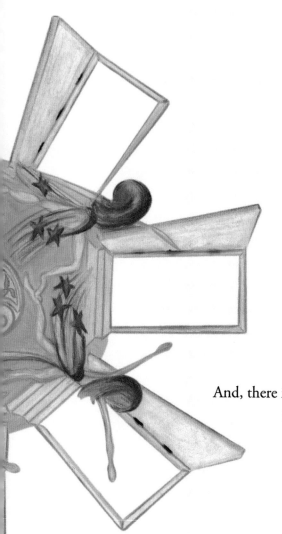

if I don't hurry
with some new worry,
I might breath
into the space,
and see what takes place.

And, there is a moment like a summer breeze:
I walk on air as it opens the doors.
The moment is gone.
But,
the next is here
and then there are more
moments like these
when I am one
with the air and the sea.

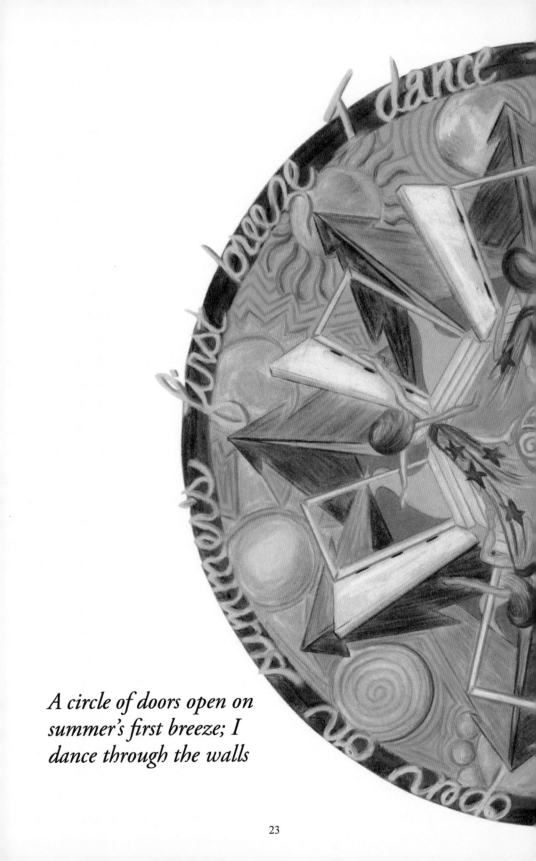

A circle of doors open on summer's first breeze; I dance through the walls

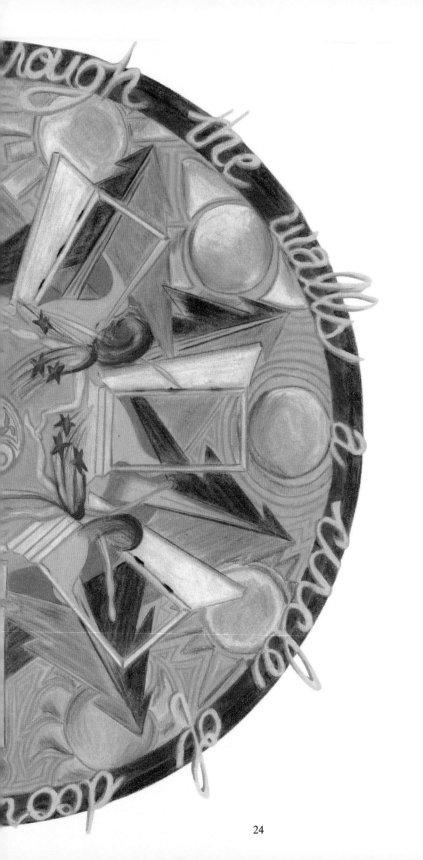

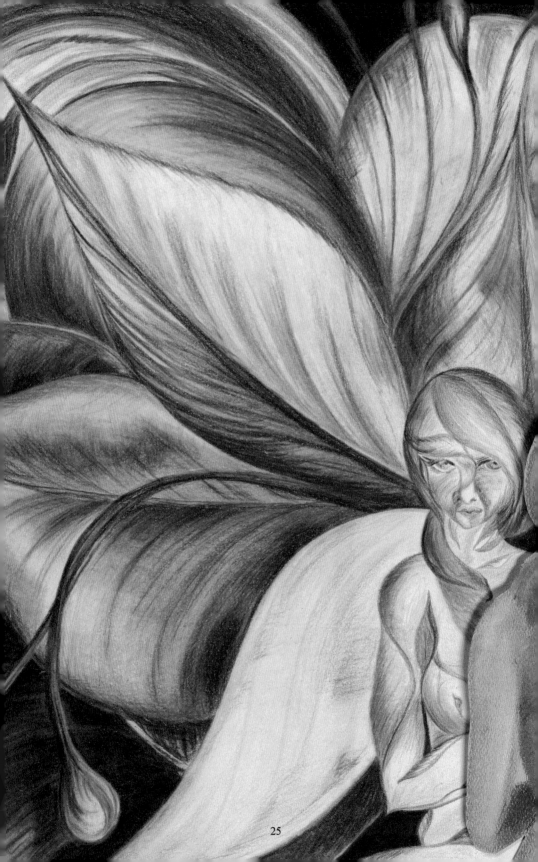

Beyond

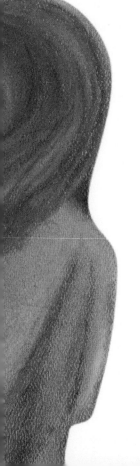

Move the body through asana,
let asana move the body then listen
as the movement stirs you, touches you deeply.

Be with the prana,
let the prana be you, then release
control of the breath, trust it, and float beyond...

... to where you might step into the sky
and dance with the stars
or be a bright star or become a star's light

... to where you might breath in the ocean
and swim with a dolphin
or be a dolphin or become the current in the sea

... to where you might walk through walls
and see beyond dimensions
or be an ageless soul or become timeless and free.

And, when you return from the journey,
to the breath, to the body what you found
might be here waiting patiently to be.

Summer Solstice

Under the orange sun
they danced
with butterflies
painting flowers
across a canvass of wheat

In sparkling waters
they swam
with dolphins
spinning air and sea
into a swirl of sky blue

Across great rivers
they ran
with pink salmon
and skipped stones
in sunlit pools of reflection

Deep in the forest
they played
hide and seek
with green shadows
beneath flickering lights of leaves

Tomorrow there's work and sleep
but today there's the dancing and playing of the longest day

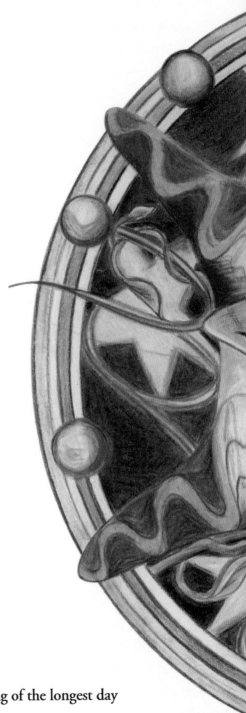

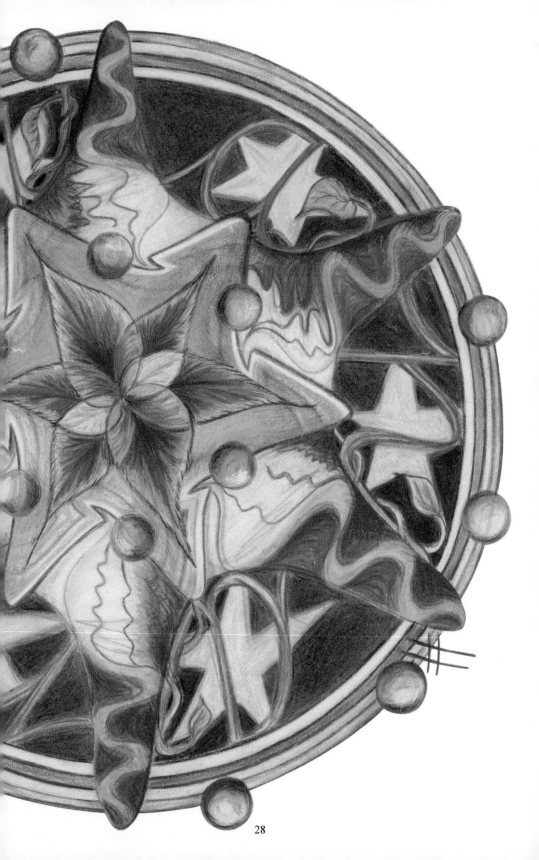

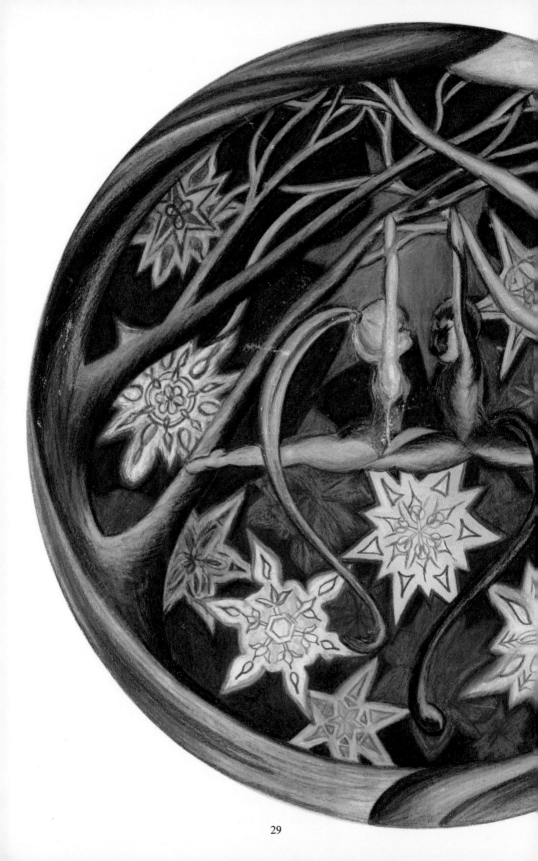

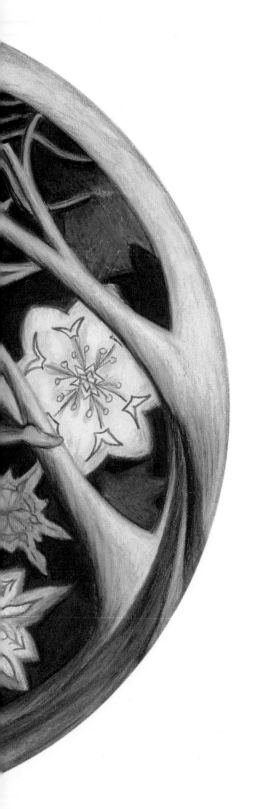

Winter Solstice

Glorious golden sunlight
a star burning bright
we celebrate it rising and setting
as it inspires our practical creativity;
we go out and work and play.

Magical silver moonlight
reflecting sun's light
we celebrate it waxing and waning
as it inspires emotional creativity;
we write songs and poetry.

Glorious magical you
go inside tonight
and celebrate winter's solstice day
for you are inspiration and creativity.
You shine bright. You reflect light.

That Perfect Edge

Where is that edge,
that perfect edge?
I ask for that is where i want to go

... where I shine like a star
while knowing I cast a shadow

... where I soar with the wind
never abandoning home

... where I float free in the clouds
keeping both feet on the ground

... where I shape tomorrow
being present with today

... and know the difference
between challenge and pain

Where is that edge,
that perfect edge?

I ask for that is where I want to go

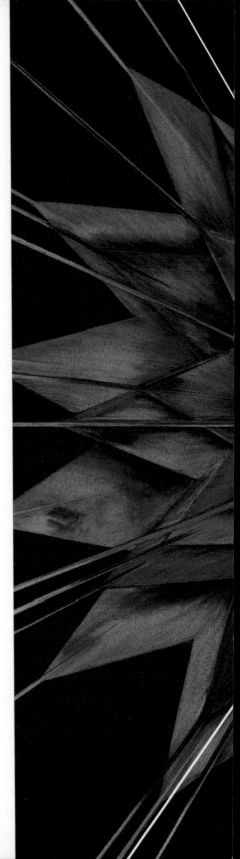

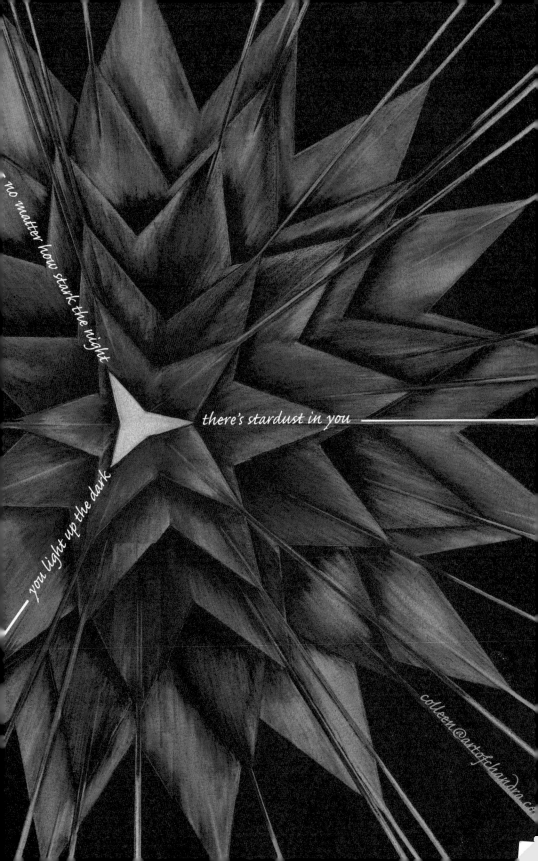

no matter how stark the night

there's stardust in you

you light up the dark

colleen@artofchandra.co

CONTENTS

PREFACE

IN this story I have followed the narrative of Josephus, making many omissions but no other change of importance. It did not fall within the scope of my work to estimate his veracity and trustworthiness; but I may here say that a close acquaintance with his history will not incline the reader to put much confidence in his narrative on any point where interest or vanity may have tempted him to depart from the truth. In one matter, which is of such interest and importance that an account of it may be given here, he seems to have deliberately falsified history. The ingenuity of a German critic, Jacob von Bernays, detected in the Chronicle of Sulpicius Severus (a Christian writer, A.D. 350?420) a very slightly disguised quotation from one of the lost books of the History of Tacitus. The passage may be thus translated.

"Titus is said to have called a council of war, and then put to it the question whether he ought to destroy so grand a structure as the Temple. Some thought that a sacred building, more famous than any that stood upon the earth, ought not to be destroyed. If it were preserved, it would be a proof of Roman moderation; if destroyed, it would brand the Empire for ever with the stigma of cruelty. On the other hand there were some, and among these Titus himself, who considered that the destruction of the Temple was an absolute necessity, if there was to be a complete eradication of the Jewish and Christian religions. These superstitions, opposed as they were to each other, had sprung from the same origin; the Christians had come forth from among the Jews; remove the root and the stem would speedily perish."

In the interest, doubtless, of his Imperial patrons, the family of Vespasian, Josephus represents the destruction of the Temple as having been accomplished against the will of Titus.

I have to express my obligations to Dean Milman's *History of the Jews*, and to the article, "Jerusalem," by Mr. Ferguson, in the *Dictionary of the Bible*. A.J.C.

OF THE BEGINNINGS OF THE JEWISH WAR

IN the fourteenth year of Nero Cæsar, Gessius Florus came down into the province of Judæa to be Governor in the room of Albinus. This Albinus had been evil spoken of for his greed and wrongdoing, but Florus far surpassed him in wickedness; for indeed he plundered whole cities and regions, nor did he refuse any man licence to rob his neighbours if only he might obtain for himself a share of the spoil.

In the beginning of the second year of Florus, Cestius Gallus, Proconsul of Syria, came to Jerusalem at the Feast of the Passover. And when the people thronged about him, making loud outcry against Florus, and praying that he would help them, Florus, who was standing at his right hand, mocked them. Nevertheless Cestius spake them fair, promising that he would speak for them to Florus, that he might deal more mercifully with them in time to come. And indeed Florus, going with him as far as Cæsarea, made many promises that he would behave himself more mercifully. Yet had he resolved in his heart that he would multiply his cruelties, that so he might drive the people into war. For he knew that, if there should be peace, the people would accuse him of his misdeeds to the Emperor, but that if there should be war, there would be no thought or remembrance of such things. Having, therefore, this purpose in his heart, he sent messengers to take seventeen talents out of the treasury of the Temple, pretending that the Emperor had need of them. But when the messengers showed their errand, immediately the whole City was in an uproar, the multitude of the people rushing to the Temple, and crying out against the tyranny of Florus. Some also of the young men went about with a basket, asking alms for the Governor as though he were a beggar. Florus, so soon as he heard these things, marched to Jerusalem with an army of horse and foot. And when the people came forth to meet him, for they would fain have pacified him, he repulsed them with violence, and commanded his soldiers to disperse the crowd. And the next day, sitting on the seat of judgment, he called before him the chief men of the City and bade them deliver up to him them that had been their leaders in the tumult, and them that had insulted him. But when he found that the guilty were not given up to him, for indeed all were guilty, not heeding the excuses and entreaties of the multitude, he gave over to his soldiers the Upper City to plunder, bidding them also slay whomsoever they might meet; which thing they did so zealously that all Jerusalem was filled with robbery and murder. Also Florus seized men of renown in the City, of whom some were Roman knights, and commanded that they should be shamefully beaten before his judgment seat, and afterwards crucified.

Now it chanced that in these days Berenice, sister to King Agrippa, was in Jerusalem, who being greatly troubled at the doings of the soldiers, sent certain of her bodyguard and captains many times to Florus, entreating him that he would have mercy upon the people. But Florus paid no heed to them; nay, when the Queen went herself and stood barefooted before his tribunal, neither he nor his soldiers regarded her, but put the prisoners to the torture, and slew them even before her eyes; and doubtless they would have slain her also, but that she escaped with her guard into the palace, and there abode for that night in great fear of death.

The next day the multitude of the people were gathered together in the market- place of the Upper City, lamenting over them that had been slain, and crying out against Florus. Nevertheless when the princes and the priests besought them that they would give no occasion to the Governor, they went peacefully to their homes. But he, desiring to stir up strife, sent to the chief men of the City, and said to them:?"If ye now be earnest for peace, go forth, and meet the soldiers that are now coming to the City, and salute them as friends." But he sent privately to the centurions, commanding that the soldiers should not take any heed of the salutations of the people. And this they did; for when the people, coming forth from the City with the priests and chief men, greeted them with all friendship, they answered nothing. This stirred up great wrath in the multitude, so that they cried out against Florus; whereupon the soldiers made at them with their clubs, chasing them back to the City, and many fell under the clubs, and yet more were trampled by the crowd.

Nevertheless when Florus would have taken possession of the Temple, the people cast stones and javelins upon the soldiers from the roofs of the houses, and beat them back; also they broke down the cloisters that were between the Tower of Antony and the Temple; which when the Governor perceived, he ceased from his purpose; and in a little space he departed to Cæsarea, leaving one cohort only for a guard to the City. Afterwards he sent letters to Cestius, accusing the Jews, and laying to their charge the very things which he had himself done against them; which letters when Cestius had read, he sent one of his captains to Jerusalem to inquire into the truth of these matters. And when this man was come he went through the whole City, beginning at Siloam, taking with him one attendant only?for the chief of the people had persuaded him, through King Agrippa, that he should do this. And when he had seen that the people were peaceably disposed, he went up to the Temple, in which place many were assembled. And having praised them and exhorted them to live quietly, he returned to Cestius.

But the chief of the people took counsel with King Agrippa, whether they should send orators to accuse Florus before Cæsar. This the King liked not, but was minded rather to exhort the people that they should submit themselves to the Romans. The multitude, therefore, being assembled on the terrace, Agrippa stood forth and spake to them many words concerning the power and greatness of the Romans, and how that they were now masters of the whole world, and persuaded them that they should submit themselves quietly. And when he had made an end of speaking, he lifted up his voice and wept, as also did Queen Berenice his sister. Thereat the people were much moved; and they cried out, "We war not against the Romans, but against Florus, for the wrong that he hath done to us. To this King Agrippa made answer, "Not so, if one look to deeds rather than to words. Your tribute ye have not paid, and ye have broken down the cloisters between the Tower of Antony and the Temple. These things ye have not done against Florus, but against Cæsar. Do ye therefore pay the tribute and build again the cloisters."

In these things the people hearkened unto the King, for they began to build the cloisters, and paid also to them that were appointed to this office what was wanting of the tribute, even forty talents. But when the King would have them render obedience to Florus, till there should come down another Governor in his room, the people reviled him, and bade him depart forthwith from the City, and some even cast stones at him. So Agrippa departed to his own kingdom.

After no long space the Jews openly rebelled against the Romans. A certain Eleazar, the son of Ananias, persuaded the people that it should not thenceforth be lawful to receive any offerings from strangers. And this was indeed the beginning of war, for they rejected the offerings of Cæsar. Then the chief men, when they had sought to turn the people from their purpose but had prevailed nothing, sent messengers to Florus and to Agrippa that they should send soldiers to Jerusalem, for that now there was a manifest rebellion. Florus, indeed, was well pleased that it should be so, and took no heed; but Agrippa sent three thousand horsemen, by whose help the chief men took possession of the Upper City. On the other hand, Eleazar and the rebels occupied the Temple. For seven days these fought against each other, and neither had the upper hand. But on the eighth day, being the festival of Wood- carrying (for on a certain day every man of the Jews was wont to bring wood for the fire upon the altar), certain of the people that are called Zealots came into the Temple. Then the rebels drove the soldiers of the King out of the Upper City, and burnt the house of Ananias, the high priest, and the palaces of the King and of the Queen, and the books in which were written the names of such as owed aught to the money-lenders. The next day they also took the Tower of Antony, and slew them that kept it; and afterwards they laid siege to the palace of Herod. And when they had assailed this for certain days but could not take it, they made a covenant with the soldiers of the King that these should come forth and suffer no injury; but with the Romans that were in the palace they would make no agreement. These, therefore, fled into the towers, for Herod had built three, the names whereof were Hippicos and Phasælis and Mariamne. But, after awhile, being reduced to great straits, they surrendered themselves, under promise from the rebels that no man should be put to death. Nevertheless so soon as they had come forth and had laid down their arms, for this also had been agreed, the rebels fell upon them and slew them all, save Metilius, their captain, for him they spared when he had promised that he would receive circumcision. And this great wickedness was wrought upon the Sabbath day.

OF THE DOINGS OF CESTIUS

WHEN tidings of these things were brought to Cestius it seemed good to him to march against the rebels. Wherefore he gathered together an army, taking the twelfth legion and auxiliaries, both horse and foot, and twelve thousand men from the three kings, to wit, Antiochus and Agrippa and Sohemus, of which twelve thousand the half were archers; and besides, many came of their own accord from the cities round about, who, though they knew but little of war, were full of zeal and hatred against the Jews; with Cestius was King Agrippa, who was a guide to the army, and also furnished it with food and with fodder for the horses.

Cestius, having burned certain cities on his way, and put their inhabitants to the sword, came near to Jerusalem, and began to pitch his camp at Gabao, which is distant six miles or thereabouts from the City. But when the Jews heard that the enemy was now approaching, they left keeping their feast and made haste to meet them; nor did they make any account of the Sabbath, though on this day they are wont to do no manner of work. Being thus very bold, by reason of their numbers, and full of courage and zeal, they fell, without keeping any order, upon the Romans; nay, so fierce were they that they broke through the line, making a great slaughter; and but that the horsemen came to the help of such as stood firm, with such also of the infantry as were not over-weary with their march, it had gone hard that day with Cestius and his whole army. Of the Romans there fell five hundred and fifteen; but of the Jews twenty-and-two only. After this the Jews went back to the City, and Cestius remained in the place for three days, the Jews watching him to see what he would do.

Then King Agrippa, seeing that the Romans were in no small danger from the multitude that was gathered in the hill country round about, judged it to be expedient to send yet again ambassadors to the Jews, who should promise to them in the name of Cestius pardon for that which was past, and peace for the time to come. For he hoped that some at the least would hearken to these words, and that so there would be made a division among them. And this, indeed, the rebels feared, for they set on the ambassadors or ever they had spoken a word, and slew one and wounded the other; and when some of the people showed indignation at such doings they drove them back to the City with clubs and stones.

When Cestius saw that they were thus divided among themselves he fell upon them with his whole army, and driving them before him, pursued them to Jerusalem. And having pitched his camp at Scopus, which is distant seven furlongs from the City, he remained quiet for three days, for he hoped, it would seem, that the inhabitants would surrender themselves to him; only during these days he sent to gather provisions from the villages that were round about. On the fourth day he et his army in array and marched into the City. Nor did the rebels seek to hinder him; for being astonished at the strength and good order of the Romans, they fled from the outer parts of the City and betook themselves to the Temple and fortified places. Then Cestius, having burned certain parts of the suburbs, came to the Upper City, and pitched his camp over against Herod's palace; and doubtless, if he had so willed, he might have conquered the rebels forthwith and so put an end to the war; but one Priscus, that was second to him in command, and certain of the captains of the horsemen, having been bribed with money by Florus, persuaded him that he should not attack the rebels. And so the war was prolonged to the utter destruction of the City. Also Ananias, the son of Jonathan, and other of the chief men of the City, had conference with him, promising that they would open the gates; trusting to whom, he sat still and did nothing. But the rebels getting a knowledge of this purpose of Ananias and his companions, cast them down from the walls, and dispersed all such as favoured them.

Cestius seeing this, gave command to the army that they should assail the Temple and the palace; and this they did for five days, but prevailed nothing. But on the sixth day Cestius, taking with him certain picked men of the legion, and archers, with them attacked the Temple from the north. These also at the first were driven back, but afterwards making a tortoise of their shields, they came close to the walls without suffering any damage and were about to put fire to the gate of the Temple. Now the manner of making a tortoise is this. They that are in the front set their shields stoutly against the walls, and to these others coming close join their shields, and to these again others. These shields being closely fitted together are as the shell of a tortoise, neither can any darts pierce through them. When the rebels saw these things they were in great fear and were about to fly, and the people were made to open the gates, and to give up the whole City to Cestius. And assuredly, if he had persevered in his undertaking, all would have gone well. But doubtless it was of God that this day brought not an end to the war. For indeed Cestius, as though he knew not the fear of the rebels, nor the temper of the people, how they would willingly receive him, suddenly called back the soldiers, and though he had suffered no great loss, contrary to the expectations of all men, departed from the City. And the rebels, seeing him thus retreat, a thing beyond all their hopes, took courage, and fell upon the rear of his army, slaying many, both horse and foot. That night Cestius abode in his camp at Scopus, but the next day he went yet further from the City, giving great encouragement to the enemy, who followed after his army and slew the hindmost, casting also javelins from either side of the way. And neither did they that were in the rear of the army dare to turn against them that assailed them, fearing the great numbers of the enemy; nor did the main body drive back them that set upon them from either side of the way, for they feared to break up their order. Also the Romans were heavily armed, but the Jews lightly equipped and ready for such kind of fighting, whence it came to pass that they suffered much loss but did no harm to the enemy.

This day there were slain with others, Priscus, that commanded the sixth legion, and Longinus, the tribune, and Æmilius Jucundus, captain of a troop of horse. And so, after much toil and loss of baggage, they came to their first camp, that is to say, the camp of Gabao. There Cestius abode two days, not knowing what he should next do. But on the third day, seeing that the number of the Jews grew greater continually, and that the whole country round about was filled with the enemy, he thought it best to depart. And that his flight might be the easier, he gave command that the soldiers should leave behind them all such baggage as might hinder them in their march; also that they should slay all the mules and beasts of burden, save such as carried the arrows of the artillery?for these things they kept, not only for their own using, but also because they feared that, falling into the hands of the Jews, they should be turned against themselves. So Cestius came to Bethhoron. Now, while the Romans were in the open country, the Jews held back, but so soon as they were come to the going down of Bethhoron, where the way is narrow, they fell upon them. And some hastening to the other end of the pass kept them from going out, and others from behind drove them down the road. Nor did the whole multitude cease to shower darts upon them till they seemed, as it were, to cover the army with them. And while the foot-soldiers stood still, not knowing how they should defend themselves, the horsemen were in a worse strait. For they could not keep their ranks and move forward by reason of the javelins that were cast against them, and the rocks on either side, being very steep and such as no horses could mount, hindered them from attacking the enemy. And on the other hand were very steep places, over which there was great peril of falling. Being therefore overwhelmed with these perils, they thought no more of defending themselves, but wept and cried aloud like men that are driven to despair, while the Jews shouted aloud for joy and for fury against their adversaries. And indeed, they were within a, little of destroying both Cestius and his whole army, but that the night coming on, the Romans made their way back to Bethhoron, where the Jews, surrounding them on all sides, watched for their coming forth.

But Cestius, seeing that he could not make his way by force, devised means by which he might fly. He chose four hundred of the bravest of his soldiers, and set them on the rampart of the camp, bidding them display the standards, that so the Jews might believe the whole army to be in the camp. And when he had done this, he himself departed in silence with the rest of his army. So soon as it was morning the Jews fell upon the camp; and when they had slain the four hundred, they pursued after Cestius. But he had been marching during no small part of the night, and now that it was day made all the speed that he could, insomuch that the soldiers cast away the battering rams and the catapults, and many other implements of war, all of which things the Jews took and used afterwards against them that had left them. And when the Romans had reached Antipatris the Jews ceased from pursuing them, and returning gathered together the implements of war, and spoiled the bodies of the dead, and collected great store of plunder, and so returned, with shouts and songs, to the City. Many Romans and auxiliaries fell in this fight, to wit of infantry five thousand and three hundred, and of horsemen three hundred and eighty.

3

OF JOSEPHUS AND THE BESIEGING OF JOTAPATA

T HERE being now open war between the Romans and the Jews, these last chose men to be their leaders, both in the City and also in the provinces; and among these was Josephus, the son of Matthias, who was set over the province of Galilee.

This Josephus was of the house and lineage of Aaron. And having been carefully taught in all things that a youth should know, he had got for himself such reputation that when he was fourteen years of age the priests and doctors of the law would come to his father's house, asking him questions concerning the more difficult matters of the law. And when he was now of about sixteen years, he purposed within himself that he would make trial of all the sects that are among the Jews; and of these sects there are three, to wit, Pharisees, and Sadducees, and Essenes. Of these he got, after great labour and trouble, full knowledge; also having heard that there was a certain Banus that dwelt in the desert, who had made to himself garments from the leaves of trees, and fed on such things as grew of themselves, he joined himself to this man, and spent three years in his company. After this he came back to Jerusalem, and being now nineteen years of age, resolved to live after the tenets of the Pharisees, the which sect may be compared to the school of the Stoics among the Greek philosophers.

When he was now twenty-and-five years of age, Josephus went to Rome; and the cause of his going was this. Felix, the Governor, had sent certain priests that were friends of Josephus to answer for themselves before Cæsar, the things whereof they were accused being but of small account. And Josephus being desirous to help them (which he was the more zealous to do when he heard that they were not forgetful of the law, but had for food figs and walnuts only, lest they should be found eating things unclean), he journeyed to Rome; in which journey he was in great danger of his life: for his ship having been broken by a storm in Hadria, he and his fellows floated on pieces of the wreck for the space of a whole night, and were taken up at dawn by a ship off Cyrene, eighty only being saved out of six hundred. Being arrived in Italy, at the city of Puteoli, Josephus made acquaintance with one Aliturus, who was an actor of plays in great favour with Cæsar, and was a Jew by birth. Thus he was made known to Poppæa that was Cæsar's wife, and by her help procured that the priests his friends should be released from their bonds. Also Poppæa gave him many gifts, so that he returned with great honour to his country.

This Josephus would fain have hindered his countrymen from rebelling against the Romans; but when he could not prevail he purposed to do them such service as he could, and was set, as hath been said, over the province of Galilee, in which government he behaved himself with great wisdom and courage. But when Flavius Vespasian came down by the command of Nero into the province of Judæa and had gathered together a great army at Antioch, even sixty thousand men, Josephus judged that he could not stand against the Romans in battle. Wherefore he commanded that all the people of Galilee should fly into the fenced cities, and he himself, having with him the bravest of his soldiers, took refuge in that which was the strongest of these cities?to wit, Jotapata. At the same time he sent letters to the rulers at Jerusalem, setting forth the whole truth; in which letters he said that if they were minded to have peace with the

Romans they should make no more delay; but that if they would have war, they would do well to send to him an army, that he might be able to join battle with the enemy.

This city of Jotapata is built upon a great hill, having cliffs about it very steep and high upon every side, save the north only; and on this Josephus, when he fortified the place, had built a great wall.

So soon as Vespasian knew that Josephus was in Jotapata, he made haste to besiege it. And first he sent soldiers, both horse and foot, who should make a road for the army; for the way was very rough, such as foot-soldiers could scarcely pass over, and horsemen not at all. This the men did in the space of four days. Afterwards he sent on Placidus, one of his lieutenants, with a thousand horsemen, bidding him watch the city, lest by any means Josephus should escape. And on the next day he himself came with the rest of his army, and pitched his camp on the north side of the city, about seven furlongs from the walls. And when the Jews saw the number of his host they were not a little dismayed, nor did they dare to come forth from the walls. The Romans, being wearied from their march, attacked not the city, but they made three lines round about it, so that none might go forth. But the Jews having now no hope of safety, were minded to fight to the uttermost. The next day Vespasian attacked the city on the north side where the wall was easy of approach; and Josephus, seeing this, and fearing lest the place should be taken, rushed out against the Romans with the whole multitude of the people and drave them back from the walls. Many were slain on both sides, for the Jews fought like men that had no hope, and the Romans were ashamed to give place. And they fought through the whole day, even until nightfall. The next day also the Romans came near to the walls, and the Jews ran out against them, and the battle was yet fiercer than before; and this was done for five days without ceasing.

After this it seemed good to Vespasian and his captains to raise a bank against the city, where the wall could be approached. For this end, therefore, he caused his whole army to fetch timber for the work, and to cut stone from the hills that were hard by. Also he caused to be set up mantlets, under cover of which the bank was made, they that built it being in nowise harmed by the stones and javelins and the like, which the Jews cast upon them from the wall. When the bank was finished Vespasian set his machines of war and catapults upon it, to the number of one hundred and sixty, which threw javelins and lighted brands and stones of a great weight, so that the Jews could not stand upon the wall, nor come to any place whither the engines could reach with their shooting. Also there was a great company of archers of Arabia and slingers that ceased not to attack the city. Nevertheless, the Jews, though they were hindered from going on to the walls, ceased not to sally from the gate; and they would drag away the shelter from them that worked, and wound the men, and they would set fire to the timber. But Vespasian, perceiving that they were able to do this, and because spaces had been left in the siege-works, commanded that these should be filled in; and when this had been done, the Jews ceased from attacking them. But when the bank had been made of equal height to the walls, Josephus, perceiving that the city was now in great danger, commanded the workmen that they should build the wall higher. And when they said that they could not do this while there were cast upon them so many javelins, he contrived this defence for them. He caused raw hides of oxen to be stretched upon stakes, and these could not either be pierced through with iron nor burnt by fire. And the men, working under cover of these, both night and day, raised the wall by twenty cubits, and built also towers upon it. This the Romans were greatly troubled to see. The Jews also, taking heart, made sallies continually from the walls against them, and did them all manner of damage. Wherefore Vespasian was minded not to suffer his soldiers to fight with them any more, but rather to blockade their city, and so at last to take them for lack of food. For he thought that they must perish or yield themselves; and that at the least, if they should be wasted with hunger, they would be the less able to fight. Therefore, sitting down before the city, he waited for the end.

Now there was sufficient in Jotapata of corn and of other things that are needful for food, save salt only. But of water there was great lack, for there is no spring in the city, and the people are content to live on such rain as falleth, taking it in cisterns. Now of rain there is but little in the summer season, in the which season it so chanced that the city was besieged. And Josephus, seeing that they had plenty of other things, and that his soldiers lacked neither numbers nor courage, and desiring that the siege should be prolonged, distributed the water to the inhabitants of the city by measure. And the Romans, perceiving that this was done, for they saw the multitude come together daily for their measure of water, and indeed cast their javelins and stones among them, slaying many, were of good hope that the city must soon yield itself. But Josephus, that he might deceive them, and cast them down from this hope, commanded that they should dip garments in water and hang them over the walls, so that the water should flow down from them to the ground. And when the Romans saw this, they were troubled, for they judged that there could be no lack of that which they saw, so to be spent to no purpose. Then Vespasian, thinking that the place would never yield itself for lack of food and drink, was resolved that he would set himself forthwith to take it by force of arms. And this was the thing which the Jews chiefly desired, for it seemed better to them to perish by the sword than to die of hunger and thirst. Also Josephus devised means by which he might hold communication with his friends that were in the cities round about. He sent letters by a certain path that there was on the western side of the valley, this path being very steep, and much overgrown, so that it was the less carefully watched; and they that bare the letters crept along the ground, being covered with skins, so that any that spied them might think they were dogs. And this was done many times, till the thing was discovered by the guards.

And now Josephus, seeing that there was no hope of escape, took counsel with the chief men of the city, concerning flight. Which when the people had knowledge of, a vast multitude came about him beseeching him that he would not leave them. "For thou," they said, "art the only hope of the place; and while thou art with us all will fight bravely, but if thou depart, no one will have the heart to stand up against the Romans." Then Josephus, fearing lest he should seem to have a thought for his own safety, spake to them saying, "If I depart,

I depart for your good; for while I am here I profit you little, so long as this city is not taken, and if it be taken, then we perish together. But if I am gone from this place, then could I profit you much, stirring up war throughout the whole region of Galilee, so that the Romans must perforce give up besieging this place. But now, knowing that I am here, and being very desirous to lay hands upon me, they are all the more urgent in their attack." Nevertheless, he prevailed nothing by these words, for the old men and women and children caught him by the feet, and besought him, with many tears, that he would not leave them. Then Josephus changed his purpose, and thought no more of leaving the city, but only how he might best make war against the Romans, vexing them day and night with all manner of attacks. And when Vespasian saw that his men suffered much loss in their encounters (for they were ashamed to give way before the Jews, nor could they pursue them on account of the weight of their armour; but the Jews, being lighter-armed and of much more agility, suffered little loss), he commanded that the soldiers of the legions, being heavy-armed, should not fight any more with the Jews; but that the Arabs and Syrians, being archers and slingers, should drive them back. As for the machines of war and the catapults, they never were quiet. Yet the Jews ceased not to give battle with the besiegers, sparing neither limb nor life.

Vespasian, seeing that he was himself in a manner besieged, for the Jews assailed him continually, judged it well to use the battering rams against the walls of the city. Now a battering ram is a great beam, like unto the mast of a ship, whereof the end is shod with iron that is of the shape of a ram's head, from which also it hath its name. This beam is hung in the middle from another beam by means of ropes, as it might be in a balance; and at either end it is rested on strong posts. This beam being first swung back with the whole strength of a great company of men, is after swung forward, and driveth the end of iron against the wall; nor is there any tower so strong, or wall of such thickness that can stand against such blows, being oftentimes repeated. Such, therefore, did Vespasian cause to be brought near to the walls; and that the working of them might not be hindered, he brought nearer also the catapults and the machines, with the slingers and archers. And when all the Jews had been driven from the walls, then they that had charge of the ram brought it up to the wall, covering it with hurdles and hides for a protection both to it and to themselves. And so soon as they drave it against the wall, the stones were shaken, and there rose a great cry from the people within, even as though the town were already taken. But Josephus, seeing that the ram was driven continually against the self-same place, and that the wall was now about to be broken down, devised means by which the violence of the attack might be diminished. He commanded that they should fill sacks with straw, and let them down in the place where the ram was about to be driven against the wall. And this they did continually, and whenever the ram was brought against the wall, then the Jews would let down the sacks of straw; and this thing made much delay and hindrance to the captains of the Romans. Then these fixed blades of iron to the end of poles and cut the ropes by which the sacks were let down. But Josephus, seeing that the ram began to work damage again, and that the wall, being for the most part newly built, was shaken by their blows, bethought him how he might help himself with fire. So he caused to be gathered together all dry wood that could be found, and making a sally with his soldiers in three divisions, set fire to the machines and siege-works of the enemy. Also they heaped on them bitumen, and pitch, and sulphur, and the fire spread itself with all the speed that can be thought, till that which it had cost the Romans the labour of many days to accomplish was destroyed in the space of one hour.

And now a certain Jew, Eleazar by name, of Sahab, in Galilee, did a thing that is worthy to be told; for, lifting up a great stone in his hands, he threw it down from the wall upon the ram so mightily that he brake off the head. And when he saw what he had done, he leapt down from the wall, and caught up the head in his hands and carried it to the wall. And though all the archers shot at him, so that their arrows stuck in his body, he heeded them not at all, but climbed the wall, and so at last, holding the ram's head in his arms, fell down overcome with weakness.

After this, Josephus and they that were with him set upon the machines and siege-works of the fifth and tenth legions?for this last had fled from its place?and burned them with fire. Nevertheless, before nightfall, the Romans brought another battering ram against that part of the wall which had been shaken at the first. Now it befell that one of them that defended the wall cast his javelin at Vespasian and smote him and wounded him; and though the wound was a small thing (for the javelin was cast from afar, and its force was spent), yet were the Romans much troubled, and especially Titus, his son. But Vespasian, making light of the pain of his wound, showed himself to the army that he was yet alive. And all the soldiers were yet more eager than before to quit themselves bravely, for they thought it shame if they should not take vengeance for the hurt which the Emperor had suffered.

Nevertheless, for all the violence of their enemies, Josephus and his soldiers stood yet upon the wall, seeking to drive back, with lighted torches and javelins and stones, them that used the battering rams. But they prevailed little or not at all; for they could not see them at whom they cast their missiles, yet could themselves be seen very plainly. For the night was as the day, by reason of the many fires that were burning, and they that stood upon the wall were manifest, nor, seeing that the machines were a long way off, could they avoid the bolts. Many indeed were slain by the darts and arrows that were cast by the artillery, and as for the stones from the catapults, they brake off the battlements of the walls and the corners of the towers. And the plying of the machines made a horrible loud noise, as also did the hissing of the stones as they flew by. These indeed were cast forth with such strength as can scarcely be believed. One that stood by Josephus on the wall was smitten by a stone, so that his head was driven, as it had been a bullet from a sling, to the length of three furlongs. And all the while there rose up from the city a great wailing of women, and from the wall the groanings of them that were wounded. Truly a man could not see or hear anything more horrible than the things which the people of Jotapata saw that night. And in the morning the wall gave way. Nevertheless Josephus and his men made up the breach as best they were able.

The next day, after that the army had rested itself and taken some food, Vespasian commanded that they should attack the city. And first he bade the bravest of his horsemen dismount; these he set in three troops at the place where the wall had been broken down. They were altogether clad in armour, and had in their hands long pikes, and it was commanded them that they should mount the breach so soon as the machine that was made for that end should be fixed. Behind these he set the best of the foot-soldiers, and behind these again the archers and slingers and them that had charge of the artillery. And on the hills about the city he set the remainder of his horsemen that none might escape when it should be taken. Others also carried scaling ladders, which they should put to the wall where it was not broken, that so some of the Jews might be called away from the defending of the breach. When Josephus perceived this he set at these parts of the wall the old men and them that were the weakest and the most wearied of his soldiers; but at the breach he set the bravest and strongest; and before all he chose six men, of whom he himself was one. To these he said, "Shut your ears against the shouting of these men; and as for their missiles, kneel upon your knees, and holding your shields over your heads, so hide yourselves till the archers have spent their arrows. But when those that ye see seek to mount the breach, then quit yourselves like men, for ye have not so much to fight for a country that yet liveth, but to avenge one that is dead. Also think within yourselves how they will slay them that are dear to you, and satisfy your wrath against them." As for the women, Josephus bade them shut themselves up in their houses, lest their crying and wailing should break the hearts of the men.

And now the trumpeters blew their trumpets, and the army shouted; and the archers and slingers sent forth a great shower of arrows and bullets, so that the day was darkened. But they that stood by Josephus, remembering the words that he had spoken to them, shut their ears against the shouting, and covered their bodies with their shields; and when the horsemen would have mounted the breach, they ran upon them with great fury. Then were many valiant deeds done on both sides; but at the last the Romans (for there were always those that came into the places of such as were wounded or slain, but the Jews had not), joining themselves closely together, and holding their shields over their heads, so advanced, and drave the Jews back from the breach.

Then Josephus, being in a great strait (when men are wont to be best at devising that which is needful), commanded that they should pour hot oil on the shields of the Romans. Of this the Jews had a plentiful store, and when they poured it down upon the Romans, these cried aloud for the pain of the burning, and brake their order, and fell back from the wall, for the oil crept under the armour from their heads even unto their feet, and consumed them even like fire; and the nature of oil is that it is easily kindled but hardly quenched.

Also the Jews used another device against them who would mount by the gangways on to the breach of the wall. They boiled a certain herb, and poured the water upon the planks of the gangways, whereby these were made so slippery that no man could stand firm upon them, but all fell, whether they sought to ascend or to descend. And when they fell the Jews cast their javelins and wounded many; so that in the end the Romans ceased from their undertaking, having had not a few slain and many wounded. Of the Jews there were slain six in all, but the number of the wounded was three hundred.

For all this the Romans lost not heart, but were rather kindled to greater wrath. Then Vespasian commanded that the bank should be made higher than before, and that there should be built upon it three towers of fifty feet in height. These towers were cased all about with iron; and this was done both that it might be the more difficult to overthrow them by reason of their weight, and also that they might not be consumed with fire. In these towers he set slingers and archers, and artillery also of the lighter sort, who themselves not being seen by reason of the great height of the tower, could yet look down upon them that defended the wall.

These then seeing that they could not escape the things that were cast upon them, nor yet cast back again others upon the enemy, and could not do any hurt to the towers (for that they were cased with iron), were driven to leave the walls; only when any sought to get footing upon them they would run out against them.

In these days, while the men of Jotapata were much troubled about their own affairs, there came tidings how that the Romans had taken the city of Joppa, and had slain all the inhabitants thereof with the sword. Also they heard that a great multitude of the Samaritans had been slain on Mount Gerizim, whither they had gathered themselves together.

On the forty-and-seventh day from the beginning of the siege there went a certain runaway to the camp to Vespasian, and showed him the whole truth, how it fared with them that were in the city, how that they were worn out with watching and fighting, and also how they might easily he taken, if he would use craft with them. For he said that at the last watch of the night, having it seemed some respite from their troubles, they were wont to take some rest, and that if he would attack the wall at that time, he would find the guards sleeping. Vespasian, indeed, doubted whether the man was speaking truth, for he knew that the Jews were, for the most part, faithful to each other, and that they could not be driven, even by the greatest torments, to betray that which they knew. Notwithstanding, thinking that even if the man spake falsely he should not receive damage, he commanded that the wall should be assailed.

Therefore, at the last watch of the night there went a company of men to the wall, who climbed on to the top; and they that stood first on the wall were Titus and another, a centurion, Domitius Sabinus by name. They found the watch sleeping, as had been told them; and when they had slain the men they went down without let into the city. Afterwards the gate being opened, the soldiers came in. And first they took possession of the citadel, and afterwards went to and fro through the city. And though the day had now dawned, yet did not the Jews know what had befallen them, for they were very weary and heavy with sleep; and also the sight of those that were awake was hindered by a great mist that chanced to prevail over the city. Nor did they understand the matter till the whole army of the Romans was in the city. These, indeed, remembering what things they had suffered in the siege for now nigh upon fifty days, had no mercy upon any. Many also of the bravest of the Jews, seeing that they could not prevail even to the avenging of themselves upon the enemy, slew themselves with their own hands. And, indeed, the Romans had that day taken the city, nor had had so much as one man slain, but for this that shall now be told. One of them that had fled into the caves that were in the city (and many had so fled) cried to a certain Antonius that he should stretch out his right hand to him, helping him to climb out of the cave. Which when Antonius had done, the other smote him from below with the spear in the groin and slew him.

All the men that were found in the city did Vespasian and the Romans slay; and the women and the children they sold into captivity. As for the city, Vespasian commanded that it should be utterly destroyed.

4

OF THE MARVELLOUS ESCAPE OF
JOSEPHUS, AND OF THE WAR IN GALILEE

S O soon as the Romans had taken the city, they began to search for Josephus, against whom they had especial wrath; also Vespasian much desired that he should be taken. Now Josephus, by the help of God, had passed through the midst of the enemy, and had leapt down into a certain deep well, out of the side of which there was a great cavern. Here he found forty of the chief men of the city that had hidden themselves, having a store of provisions such as would suffice for many days. That day indeed he lay in this place, but at night he went forth, seeking for some way of flight, if such there might be. But seeing that all the place was watched with exceeding care (which indeed the Romans did on his account), he descended again into the cave, and so lay hid for two days. But on the third day, a certain woman that had been in the place, going forth, revealed the whole matter to Vespasian. And he straightway sent two tribunes to Josephus, who coming to the place, were earnest with him that he should give himself up, promising that his life should be granted to him. But they did not persuade him, when he considered with himself what grievous harm he had done to them in the days of the siege. Then Vespasian sent a third tribune also, one Nicanor, that in former time had been a friend to Josephus. This Nicanor, coming to him, set forth how that the Romans were ever merciful to them whom they had subdued, and how that the generals had admiration rather than hatred for him by reason of his valour, and that it was the purpose of the Emperor not to slay him, which indeed he could do without making conditions, but to save him alive, being so brave a man. But while Josephus doubted what he should do, for the words of Nicanor were weighty, the soldiers, growing impatient, would have thrown fire into the cave; but their captain hindered them, desiring above all things to take Josephus alive. Then as he considered the promises of the Emperor on the one hand, and the threatenings of the soldiers on the other, there came into his mind the remembrance of certain dreams that he had dreamed, wherein God had showed him beforehand what great trouble would befall the nation of the Jews, and also what should be the fortune of the Emperor of Rome. Now Josephus was well skilled in the interpretation of dreams; and also he had good knowledge of the prophecies of the holy books, seeing that he was a priest, and that his forefathers had been priests before him. Considering these things, therefore, he prayed in secret to God, saying, "Since it hath seemed good to Thee to bring down the nation of the Jews, and since Thou hast given power over the earth to these Romans, and also hast chosen me that I might prophesy things to come, I yield myself to these my enemies, and refuse not to live. But I call Thee to witness that I go not as a traitor, but as Thy servant."

When he had thus prayed, he prepared to come forth; but when the Jews that were in the cave with him perceived what he was about to do they came round about him, clamouring with these words: "Canst thou endure, O Josephus, for love of life to be a slave? How quickly hast thou forgotten thy own words and those whom thou didst persuade to die for freedom's sake! And thinkest thou that they will suffer thee to live to whom thou hast done so much hurt? But, however this may be, though thou be blinded with the glory of the Romans, yet will we take care for the honour of our country. Here then we offer thee a sword and a hand that shall use it against thee. And if thou diest willingly, then thou art still our leader: but if unwillingly, then thou art a traitor." And as they said these words, they pointed their swords at him, affirming that they would assuredly slay him if he should yield himself, to the Romans.

Then Josephus spake to them, seeking to show them that he did well in yielding himself to the Romans; for that though it was an honourable thing for a man to die for his country, yet he should die in battle, and not by his own hand. "For will not God," he said, "be wroth, if a man despise the gift which He has given him, even the gift of life? For whomsoever squandereth or loseth that which is put into his charge, he is counted as wicked and traitorous. How then shall God punish him who shall wilfully destroy that thing which He hath committed unto him?"

With these and many like words Josephus would fain have persuaded them that they should not slay one another. But they, as men that had their ears deafened by very many sounds, were greatly wroth with Josephus, and ran upon him with their swords, reviling him for his cowardice. Then Josephus called every one by name; and at some he looked sternly as a captain might do, and another he would take by the hand, and another he would beseech with many prayers, turning, as a wild beast when it is surrounded by the pursuers, to each one as he came near. So because they had not altogether forgotten what reverence they had had for him in former days, they let go their swords, waiting for what he should say. Then, when he had committed himself to God, he said, "Since ye are resolved to die, let us cast lots how we shall slay one another, so that each man may die, when he shall have drawn the lot, by the hand of his companion. So shall we all die, yet shall no man slay himself." To these words they all consented, and the lots were drawn. Then he to whom the lot first fell out willingly offered his neck to him that was next to him; for they were persuaded that their captain also would die with them, and they judged it better to die in company of Josephus than to live without him. And in the end?but whether this was of chance or of the ordering of God, cannot be said?Josephus was left alive with one other; and when these two were about to draw the lot, Josephus persuaded him that he should live, wishing neither himself to die nor to slay his companion.

Then did Nicanor lead Josephus to Vespasian; and all the Romans were gathered together to see him, so that there was a great commotion, some shouting for joy that he was taken, and some threatening him, and many pressing forward to look upon him. Of them that were furthest from him, many cried out that he should be put to death, but such as stood close to him remembered the great deeds that he had done; and as for the captains, even such as had before been full of wrath against him, when they looked upon him had compassion on him. And chiefly Titus, being of a generous temper, was well inclined to him, remembering how bravely he had borne himself in battle, and yet was now a prisoner in the hands of his enemies, and considering how great is the power of fortune, and what changes befall men in war, and how mutable are the affairs of men. Now Titus had great power with his father, and was instant with him that he would save Josephus alive. Nevertheless, Vespasian commanded that he should be kept with all care, being minded to send him to Nero forthwith.

When Josephus knew that he had this purpose in his heart, he said that he would gladly speak a few words with him in private. Therefore when all had departed from him, save Titus and two of his friends only, Josephus spake, saying:?"I have great things to tell thee, O Vespasian. For indeed, have I not been sent to thee of God? Thou knowest the custom of the Jews, and how it becometh the captain of a host to die. Dost thou send me to Nero? Know that thou shalt be Emperor, thou, and thy son after thee. Bind me therefore, and keep me, to see whether my words be true or no." Now Vespasian did not believe the words of Josephus, thinking that he had feigned them for the saving of his own life. But afterwards he changed his mind, for indeed God had put the thought of this very thing into his heart, and had also showed him beforehand by many signs of the things that were to come. And when one of the friends of Vespasian said:?"I marvel much, Josephus, why thou didst not prophesy to the men of Jotapata, how their city should be taken, and how thou shouldest thyself be led into captivity," Josephus answered him, saying:?"Nay, but I did prophesy to the men of Jotapata that after forty-and-seven days their city should be taken, and also that I should myself be taken prisoner by the Romans." When Vespasian made inquiry of the captives he heard that this was indeed the truth; and after this he believed the words of Josephus. And though he set him not free from his chains, yet did he give him change of raiment and other gifts, and had him in great honour; and in all these things Titus was his friend.

After these things the other cities of Galilee that yet remained to the Jews were taken, as Joppa, and Tarichæa, and Gamala. Tiberias, indeed, that is by the Lake of Galilee, yielded itself to the Romans; and Vespasian, though he destroyed the other cities and put their inhabitants, for the most part, to the sword, had mercy upon the inhabitants of Tiberias, for he knew that this would be well pleasing to King Agrippa.

On this Lake Galilee there was fought a great battle of ships, between the Romans and certain of the inhabitants that had fled from Tarichæa when they saw that it was now about to be taken. For Vespasian, when he had taken the city, put into ships so many of his soldiers as he thought sufficient for the purpose, and sent them against the men of Tarichæa. These indeed were in a great strait, for they could not disembark from their boats on to the land, inasmuch as there was no place that was not in the power of the enemy, nor could they meet the Romans in battle, for their boats were small and light, and such as could not contend against ships of war. Nevertheless, rowing round the ships, they cast stones and javelins at them from afar; and sometimes they would come close and strike at them. But they did hurt to themselves rather than to their enemies. For the stones were of no avail, being cast at men that were clothed in armour, but they were themselves grievously wounded by the javelins of the Romans; and such as dared to come near were struck down before they could do anything, and oftentimes were sunk, together with their vessels. Many did the Romans slay with their pikes, and many also they slew with swords, and some they took alive in their boats. And if one of them that was overthrown into the water lifted up his head, an arrow would smite him, or he would be taken by them that were in the ships; and if, in their despair, the men swam to the ships and laid hold of them, the Romans would cut off their hands or their heads. Many, therefore, were slain or taken in the midst of the water, and those that sought to escape to the land were slain by the Romans so soon as they leapt out of their boats. And the whole lake was filled with blood and with dead bodies of men, for none escaped.

5

OF THE TROUBLES IN JERUSALEM

IN the meantime, while these things came to pass in the land of Galilee, there were great troubles in the City of Jerusalem. For whereas the princes and the people had chosen Ananus, the High Priest, to be their ruler, a certain Eleazar, the son of Simon, prevailed against him; and this he did by his subtlety and by help of the abundance of the money which he had?for he had laid hold of that which Cestius the Roman was carrying with him for the wages of his soldiers, and of that which was in the public treasury. Now Ananus, and they that were with him, made great preparation of arms and instruments of war, and strengthened the walls, as though they would defend the City against the Romans. This they did to please the people, but their purpose was to cease from these preparations after a while, and to turn the hearts of the Zealots?for so men called the rebels?to moderation and prudence. But this they could not do.

After these things there came to Jerusalem one John, the son of Levi, who was also called John of Gischala. This man had fled by night from Gischala, in which city he had fought against the Romans, after that all the rest of the land of Galilee had been subdued. And when the people had gone forth to meet him and his companions,

inquiring how it had fared with them, though it was manifest that the
men had fled with all the speed they might, so quickly did they fetch
their breath, yet they talked bravely, affirming that they had not fled
from the Romans, but were rather come to Jerusalem that they might
fight with the more advantage; "For we would not spend our lives for
nought," they said, "at Gischala and places of no account, but would
defend Jerusalem, being the chief city of our nation." And when the
people doubted what they should do, John was very urgent with
them that they should be stubborn in rebelling against the Romans,
who, he said, were now in evil case, and could not, even if they should
get themselves wings, climb the walls of Jerusalem; and besides had
had great loss in besieging the towns of Galilee, and suffered great
damage to their machines.

And now throughout all the land, and especially in Jerusalem,
was there strife between the lovers of peace and those that delighted
in war; of whom, in the end, the latter prevailed. Besides this, the
whole country was wasted by robbers, so that it seemed to the inhabitants a lighter thing to be led into captivity by the Romans than to
suffer such violence. And of these robbers not a few crept secretly
into Jerusalem?for into the City all were admitted without question?
who afterwards had no small share in bringing it to destruction, for
they caused tumult without end, and also consumed the provisions
which had sufficed for the men of war. These men, taking for their
leader Eleazar the son of Simon, filled the whole City with robbery
and slaughter. And this they did not secretly, but openly and in the
day; nor did they lay hands on common folk only, but on the great
men and princes, such as was Antipas, the treasurer of the City, who
was of the lineage of Herod. Him, and others with him, they at the
first shut up in the prison, but afterwards, fearing lest they should be
delivered by their kinsfolk, and that the people might make insurrec-
tion, they sent a certain John, the son of Dorcas, with ten swordsmen,
and slew them in the prison.

Also they set aside the law of inheritance, according to which the
chief priests were wont to be appointed, and made chief priests of
whom they would?men altogether mean and base. And for high

priest they chose one Phannias, the son of Samuel, a clownish fellow and one who knew not at all what this office of the priesthood might mean. Him they took, against his will, from his farm, and adorned with robes, as one who acts is adorned upon the stage, and sought to teach him what he should do. All this was an occasion of mirth and laughter to them, but the priests, as they stood afar off, wept to see the law despised in this fashion.

Then the high priest, Ananus, a wise man, who haply might have saved the City if the wicked had suffered him to live, called the people together to an assembly, and sought to stir them up against Simon and the Zealots, reproaching them that they suffered such wickedness to be done, none raising a hand to hinder it. "Think," he said, "how your forefathers fought many and great battles that they might be free. And ye also, why do ye now wage war against the Romans but for this same cause? Yet ye suffer yourselves to be made slaves by these robbers. And verily, if the Romans should conquer you, what could ye suffer worse or more grievous than what ye now endure at the hands of these men? For these slay them whom the Romans harmed not; and whereas the Romans went not into the Holy Place, which it is not lawful but for the priests to enter, these men, being, as they say, Jews, profane it daily. Come, therefore, and give your lives, if need be, for the honour of the Lord; and as for me, ye shall not see me hold back from danger."

With these and many like words the high priest Ananus exhorted the people. And after this he held a levy, and armed such as gave their names, and set them in order of battle. Which when the Zealots perceived they sallied forth from the Temple in great wrath and fell upon the people. And these on their side fought against the Zealots. And of the two the people were the more in number by far, but the Zealots were the better armed. But both fought with all their might, for the people judged that it were better to die than to serve these robbers, and the Zealots knew that if they were conquered they must die, and at last, as the multitude of the people increased continually, and those that were behind suffered not such as were in front to give way, the Zealots perforce gave way, and fled into the Temple, Ananus and the people following hard after them. And when, leaving the Outer Court, which is also the Court of the Gentiles, they entered into the Inner Court, and shut to the gates, Ananus judged it not wise to force the place; for the Zealots were throwing javelins and the like from above; and also he would not bring the people into the Court, being not yet purified from blood. Nevertheless, he set six thousand men in the cloister of the Temple to watch it; and other six thousand to come in their places after a time. And to this service all the citizens were bound; only the wealthier sort hired poor men to stand in their stead.

Now John of Gischala was of the number of those with whom the high priest took counsel. He was a subtle man, and one who sought favour for himself; and though he seemed to be zealous for the people, sitting in the council by day and visiting the watchers by night, yet did he betray everything to the Zealots. Which when Ananus began to suspect, for it was manifest that the plans were betrayed, and yet could not rid himself of John, he would have him take an oath. This the man did with all willingness, swearing that he would be zealous for the people, and would betray nothing to the enemy, but would do all that he might for their overthrow. And Ananus and they that were with him believed the man, insomuch that they sent him to treat with the Zealots for peace. But John's words, when he was come into the Temple, were altogether contrary to the purpose of them that sent him. For he said of Ananus, that he had sent messengers to Vespasian, that he should come without delay and take the City; also that he would use the pretence of purifying the Temple to assail them. "As for you," he said, "I see not how ye can either endure a siege or fight against this great multitude. Wherefore ye must either submit yourselves to Ananus, or seek help from without. And if you submit yourselves, ye know well what mercy ye may look for, remembering what things ye have done in time past against the people."

Now of this help from without, John dared not to speak openly; but his thought was of the people of Idumæa (Idumæa is the land of Edom); and Eleazar and his fellows doubted for a while what they should do; but at last it seemed good to them to call the Idumæans. Wherefore they wrote a letter, saying:?"Ananus, the high priest, having deceived the people, is ready to betray the City to the Romans; and we, having rebelled against him for freedom's sake, are besieged in the Temple, and must perish speedily unless ye come to our help and to the help of the City against the Romans." This letter they sent by two fleet runners; nor did they doubt but that the Idumæans would hearken to their words, for they are a turbulent folk, delighting in change, and hastening to a battle with as good a will as to a feast.

So soon as the chiefs of the Idumæans had read the letter and heard the words of the messengers, they gathered together an army with all speed, and sent it, even two thousand men, to Jerusalem. Now, Ananus had not perceived the going forth of the messengers; but of the coming of the Idumæans he knew beforehand. Wherefore he shut the gates of the City and set guards upon the walls. Nevertheless he purposed not to fight against them, but rather to win them over by words. For this cause he sent to them a certain Joshua, who was next to himself among the priests. This man stood upon a turret of the wall over against them, and spake to them. He reproached them that they were come to help a company of robbers against their own kinsfolk. "As to this accusation of treachery," he said, "that they bring against us, it is altogether false. For what proof have they? Can they show any letter that we have sent to the Romans? Have they laid hands on any messenger? But as for the things which they themselves have done, come into the City (though ye come not in as conquerors), and see them for yourselves. Ye will see houses desolate and mourners everywhere; yea, and the Holy Place, which the whole world worshippeth, trampled under foot of these wild beasts."

To this Simon, son of Cathlas, who was captain of the Idumæans, made reply, that he and his fellows were come to defend the Holy City against traitors and enemies, and that it was their purpose not to depart till this had been accomplished. Nevertheless many doubted whether they had done well in coming; yet being ashamed to go back without doing aught, they abode under the walls. Now, that night, there was a very grievous storm of wind and rain, with lightnings and thunderings. And the Idumæans gathered their whole company together as close as might be, and joining their shields over their heads, so kept off the rain, nor did they take much harm from it. But the Zealots were much concerned on their behalf, and took counsel together how they might help them. And some of the bolder sort would have set upon the guards of the gates. "For they are not men of war," they said, "and will without doubt give way before us. Nor will they easily gather the citizens together, by reason of the rain and wind. And indeed, if there be danger, yet must we endure it rather than see our friends perish." But the more prudent would have them gain their end by craft rather than by force. For they saw that the guard was larger than it was wont to be, and that the walls of the City were kept with the more diligence by reason of the Idumæans. And they thought that Ananus would himself see to the ordering of all things. And indeed this was his custom; but for that night he omitted it, it being so decreed that he and his fellows should perish. And so it fell out that at midnight the guards were dispersed, lying down to sleep in the porches. Then took the Zealots the sacred saws out of the Temple, and cut through the bolts of the gates; neither could the noise of the sawing be heard for the roaring of the wind and the pealing of the thunder.

So they opened the gate that was nearest to the Idumæans; and these at first were slow to enter, doubting whether this might not be some stratagem of Ananus. But when they knew who had done it, straightway they entered. Now, if they had turned to the City to attack it, doubtless they had destroyed it wholly, so furious were they. But they that had opened the gates were urgent with them that they should first deliver such as were shut up in the Temple. "For if ye do this," they said, "and scatter the guard, afterwards ye can do what ye will to the City."

So the Idumæans went up to the Temple; and when the Zealots that were within saw them come near, they sallied forth and set upon the guard. Some they slew, being not yet awaked out of sleep; but the rest caught up their arms with all speed and defended themselves.

And this they did with sufficient courage, so long as they thought that they had the Zealots only to deal with; but when they knew that the Idumæans were come into the City, many of them cast away their arms and began to weep and to lament. Notwithstanding, a few of the young men bare themselves bravely. And though their fellows in the City knew in what a strait they were, yet durst they not come to their help for fear of the Idumæans; but there was made a great crying and wailing of women. And the Idumæans and the Zealots shouted as they fought; and the noise was the more terrible by reason of the storm. The Idumæans had mercy upon none, for they are a savage folk, but slew all alike, whether they fought or prayed for mercy. And because there was no way of escape, many threw themselves down into the City below, and so perished miserably. And all the Temple was swimming with blood; and when it was day, they counted the dead bodies, and found that the number of them was eight thousand and five hundred. After this, the Idumæans turned to the City, spoiling the houses, and slaying all whom they met. And especially were they furious against Ananus the high priest and against Joshua. These they took and slew forthwith. Moreover, such was their wickedness, they cast forth the dead bodies of these holy men without burial; though the Jews are commonly so careful in this matter that they take down the dead bodies of them that are crucified, that they may bury them before the setting of the sun.

Now this slaying of Ananus may well be counted as the beginning of the destruction of the City. For he was a righteous man, and a lover of liberty, and one who set the good of the state before his own advantage. Also he was very earnest for peace, knowing that it was not possible to prevail over the Romans, and that the nation must needs perish in the war, unless they could come to some conditions of peace. Which thing doubtless had been done, if only he had lived, for he was a skilful orator and one who could persuade the people. But without doubt, because it was the pleasure of God to destroy the City that had so defiled itself, and to purge the Holy Place with fire, therefore He cut off from the people such as might have saved them.

6

OF THE FIRST COMING OF THE ROMANS

A FTER this the Zealots and the Idumæans slew a great multitude of the people. But many of the princes and of the better sort they cast into prison, hoping that so they might win them over to their own cause. Nevertheless of these prisoners not one would hearken to their persuasions; for they judged it better to die than to be numbered with those wicked men that were conspiring against their own country. So great was the fear among the people that none durst openly lament for his kinsfolk, or so much as bury them; but they wept for the dead in secret, and were careful that the enemy should not hear their groans. And at night, or even by day, if there was found a man a little bolder than his fellows, they would throw earth upon the dead bodies.

After a while they grew weary of slaughtering after this fashion, and would set up mockeries of courts and judgment seats. There was a certain Zacharias, the son of Baruch, a wealthy man and a powerful, and a lover of liberty. Him they took and brought before seventy judges whom they had chosen from the people, being men wholly without authority. And when they accused him that he sought to betray the country to the Romans and had sent messengers to Vespasian for this end, but could bring no proof or witness of what they laid against him, Zacharias, knowing that his case was desperate, spake out his mind with all freedom. And first he showed the truth about the things whereof he was accused, and proved that the charge which they laid against him was naught; and afterwards he turned against his accusers, setting forth their misdeeds in order and lamenting the ruin that they had brought to pass. When the Zealots heard these words, they cried out against him, and could scarce refrain from drawing their swords upon him, only they would fain have the trial brought to an end, that they might know how these judges would bear themselves. Nevertheless the seventy acquitted the man, choosing rather to die themselves than to condemn him to death. But when this judgment was declared all the Zealots cried out. And two of the boldest ran upon Zacharias and smote him with their swords, crying, "This is the vote we give thee; of this acquittal there can be no question." Then they threw down the dead body into the valley below. As for the judges they smote them with the flat of their swords, and drave them out of the Temple. But now the Idumæans began to repent them that they had come, and to grow weary of these ill deeds. And while they thus thought on these things, there came one of the Zealots to them and unfolded all the frauds and deceits of his fellows. "As for the betraying of the City to the Romans," he said, "we have found no proof of it, and now we had best have nothing more to do with these men; else we shall surely be counted guilty of all their misdeeds."

So the Idumæans departed; but first they set free those that lay bound in the prisons, to the number of two thousand. But when they were gone, the Zealots raged against their adversaries more furiously than before; and especially against all the better sort of the people, for they judged that they should scarcely be safe, if they left even one of them alive. The chief of them that they slew were Gorion, a man well born and of great honour, whom they hated for his freedom of speech, and Niger of Peræa, who had borne himself very bravely in battle against the Romans. This Niger they dragged through the City while he cried out against their wrongdoings, and showed the scars of his wounds. And when he found that they led him without the gates, he asked of them that they would at least give his body to his kinsfolk for burial. But even this they denied to him. Then he lifted up his voice, being at the point to die, and cried that the Romans would avenge him, and that they should suffer not war only, but hunger also and pestilence, and that they should be slain by each other's hands; all which things, for the greater punishment of these wicked men, God brought upon them.

When the Roman captains heard that there was such strife in the City, they thought to profit by it, and would have marched forthwith to assail it, saying to Vespasian, who was over the whole host, "Surely now God is on our side, seeing that our enemies have turned their hands against each other. Let us, therefore, make haste before they repent them of their folly and make peace among themselves." But Vespasian made answer, "Ye perceive not what is best for us, and are like not to true soldiers, but those who make display of their arms in the theatre; only that your display is not without peril. For if we march against their City forthwith, then shall we bring it to pass that they be reconciled to each other, and will thus turn their strength against us. But if we wait, then shall we have the fewer to deal with. Nay, it is God who is a better captain than I, for He giveth the Jews into our hands without toil or peril. Wherefore if we look to our safety, it were best to leave them to destroy themselves; and if we look to our honour, let us not suffer it to be said that we have conquered by their strife rather than by our valour."

To these words of Vespasian all the captains gave assent. And indeed it was speedily manifest that his counsel was wise; for day by day many deserted to the Romans, escaping from the Zealots; though indeed it was not an easy thing to escape, for the Zealots kept all the ways; and if one was taken he was slain forthwith as a deserter. Yet if a man had the wherewithal to bribe the guards, he was loosed, and they were only counted for traitors who had nothing which they could give. And all the streets were filled with dead bodies; nor was it permitted for the kinsfolk of the slain to bury them; but if anyone dared to do this he was punished with death. And as for those that languished in the prisons, so great was their misery that they counted the dead to be happy in comparison of themselves.

About this time there came news to Vespasian of troubles in Gaul, where indeed Vindex had revolted against Nero. And when he heard these tidings he was the more desirous to finish the war, judging that there would be great confusion throughout the world, and peril to the whole Empire; and that if he could first bring about peace in the East, there would be the less fear for Italy. Wherefore during the winter he set garrisons in such towns and villages as he had subdued, building up again much that had been destroyed. And when it was spring he set out with the greater part of his army; and so, having subdued other regions, came to Jericho, which city he found desolate, for the dwellers therein had fled to the hill country of Judæa. Here he made a camp, and others elsewhere, so that now it was not possible for any that were in Jerusalem to come out thence.

But when he was now preparing to assault the City, there came news to him from the West, which caused him to delay his purpose; for he heard that Nero was dead (having reigned thirteen years and eight days). And first he waited till he should know who had been made Emperor in Nero's stead. And when he heard that Galba had been made, he would take nothing in hand till he should have his commands; but he sent Titus, his son, to salute him, and hear from him what he should do. With Titus went also King Agrippa. But while they sailed by Cyprus they heard that Galba was dead, and that Otho was now Emperor. Then indeed Agrippa went on to Rome, but Titus sailed across to Cæsarea to his father. And Vespasian, seeing that there was such confusion in the Empire, thought the time unseasonable for making war, and so held his hand.

But, meanwhile, there came to be great troubles in Jerusalem, and these from a certain Simon, the son of Gioras, who, when Ananus was dead, conceived in his heart the hope of ruling the City, and gathered together for this end an army of wicked men. He built for himself a fort at a certain village called Nain; and in the valley of Pharos, where there are many caves, he hid away the plunder which he had taken.

After a while the Zealots, fearing the man and his counsels, for they doubted not that he had it in his mind to take the City, came out and fought against him. But they fled before him, and many were slain, and the others driven back into the City. Yet he durst not as yet attack the walls, but went back to his fort. After this he made war on the Idumæans, and laid waste their country, and took many cities therein; and afterwards, coming back, pitched his camp without Jerusalem, surrounding it with a wall; and coming out thence he slew such as would have entered the City.

Meanwhile there arose great strife in the City among those who followed John of Gischala. For such of them as were Idumæans?and there were yet many Idumæans in the City?conspired against him, either being envious of his power, or hating him for his cruelty. Then these men and those who still clave to John fought together; but though they prevailed in the battle, they doubted how this matter should turn out, for the followers of John were many and desperate, and they feared lest they should burn the City. Therefore that they might overthrow John they purposed to bring Simon, the son of Gioras, into the City. And this counsel was performed, for they sent Matthias, the high priest, and besought him, whom aforetimes they had feared, to enter the City. And this he did, making loud and boastful promises that he would set the people free from their tyrants; and the people answered with much shouting and applause. Yet when he had taken it he counted all alike for enemies, both them who had sent for him, and them against whom these would have had him fight.

This happened in the third year of the war. And straightway Simon took possession of the Upper City, and shut up John in the Temple, which also he would fain have taken. But this he could not do, for John and his men had the highest ground, and upon this they had built four great towers, on which they set their engines, with their bowmen and the slingers, so that many of Simon's men were slain.

About this time there came tidings to Vespasian that Vitellius was made Emperor, for Otho had been conquered by him. With this

Vespasian was very ill content; yet when he thought what changes and chances there are in war, and how fickle a thing is fortune, he doubted what he should do. But the soldiers were very urgent with him that he should consent to be Emperor, for they could not endure that such a one as Vitellius should rule over them. And to this after a while he consented.

Then did he begin to consider with himself that he had been called to this dignity by the providence of God. Also he remembered besides other signs, and indeed there had been many, which had portended to him this sovereignty, and also the words which Josephus had spoken to him; for while Nero was yet alive he had dared to call him Emperor. And he was astonished that the man who had done this should yet be held as a prisoner. Wherefore, calling for Mucianus and his other captains and friends, he set forth to them what great things Josephus had done, and how he had hindered him when he was besieging Jotapata, and after had prophesied to him, and how having suspected before that these prophecies were feigned, that the man might save himself thereby, he now knew that they were spoken by the inspiration of God. "Surely," he said, "it is a shameful thing that he who prophesied to me my sovereignty, and was the minister of the voice of God, should yet be held in the estate of a captive and a prisoner." Then he called for Josephus, and commanded that he should be loosed from his chains. But Titus, who stood by, said, "It is right, sire, that Josephus should be set free, not from the chains only, but from the reproach also. And this shall be if the chains be not loosed but cut asunder." For this is the custom with such as have been wrongfully bound. To this Vespasian gave consent; and one stepped forth and cut asunder his chains with an axe. Thus did the words of his prophecy bring him into good repute, and thereafter he was counted as one who might be believed when he spake of things to come.

After this Vespasian went to Antioch; and from Antioch, after a while, to Alexandria. And being at Alexandria he heard good tidings from Rome, how that Vitellius was dead, and that all received him for Emperor; and indeed there came envoys from all parts of the world to do him homage. Then he himself proposed to go to Rome; but he sent Titus, his son, to take the City of Jerusalem, and Titus, having sailed down the Nile as far as Mende, led his army thence to Cæsarea, to which place he came after a nine days' march; and there he purposed to set his army in order for the siege.

7

THE BEGINNING OF THE SIEGE

MEANWHILE the strife in the City waxed yet fiercer than before. For now Eleazar, the son of Simon, who had at the first separated the Zealots from the people, and taken possession of the Temple, began to stir himself. He made indeed as though he could not any longer endure the doings of John of Gischala, for John ceased not from shedding blood, but in sooth he was not content to be under the rule of another sect, but would have the dominion for himself. Therefore he revolted from John, and drew away not a few of the Zealots after him. With these he seized the Inner Court of the Temple. Of stores indeed they had sufficiency, for the Temple was well furnished with them; nor did they abstain from anything, as accounting it sacred. But because they were few in number they went not forth beyond the enclosure. As for John of Gischala, he was superior to Eleazar in the number of his men, but inferior in the advantage of his place; for he had the enemy above, and so could not attack them without peril, yet could not for wrath remain quiet. Wherefore though he suffered more damage than he caused to Eleazar and his fellows, yet he slackened not at all, but assailed them without ceasing; and the Temple was defiled daily with bloodshed.

As for Simon, the son of Gioras, who possessed the whole of the Upper City, and a great part of the Lower, he assailed John with the more fury, as knowing that he was being assailed by Eleazar also from above. But he was lower than John, as John was lower than Eleazar. As for John, he drove back them that assailed him from below with no great trouble, and them that were above he checked with his engines of war and artillery, for he had these in plenty, throwing stones and bullets and the like, with which he slew not the enemy only, but many also of them that came to do sacrifice in the Temple. And indeed, for all their madness and wickedness, the Zealots refused not entrance to such as would offer sacrifice, admitting the people of the land not without suspicion, but strangers freely. These then would often be slain in the midst of their sacrificing, for the stones from the artillery reached to the altar itself, so great was the force of them.

Now therefore there were three parties in the City striving with each other. And in this strife they destroyed, as though of set purpose, all that had been stored in the City for the enduring of a siege, and in other things also served the cause of the enemy. For all the space that was round about the Temple was wasted with fire, being made ready, as it were, for the ordering of an army therein; and all the wheat, excepting a little only, which had otherwise sufficed for many years, was destroyed.

And now began many, the old men especially and the women, to pray for the coming of the Romans, having indeed no other hope of deliverance. But as for escape, that was not possible to any, for all the ways were diligently guarded; and though the armed men strove with each other, yet they agreed in this, that they counted for enemies such as seemed to them to desire peace with the Romans, and slew them without mercy.

And now John of Gischala took of the consecrated timber that he might make thereof engines of war. For before this the priests and the people had thought to build the Temple higher by twenty cubits; and for this end King Agrippa had caused that there should be brought down from Mount Lebanon great beams, suitable for the work, doing this with great cost of money and with much labour. And these beams were of marvellous size and beauty; and John, seeing that they were of suitable length for his purpose, built of them great towers on the west side of the Temple, seeking thus to be on a level with them that assailed him from above.

By the help of these towers he hoped that he should prevail over his enemies; nor did he heed at all that the timber was consecrated. Yet did God show him that his labour was in vain; for before that any man set foot in the towers the Romans came upon the City. For by this time Titus had set out from Cæsarea; and part of his army he had with him, and to part he had given commandment that they should meet him at Jerusalem. Three legions he had under him with which his father Vespasian had laid waste the whole land of Judæa; he had the twelfth also, which legion had suffered defeat under Cestius, and having always been renowned for courage, was now the more eager to avenge itself upon the Jews. The fifth legion also was coming to meet him, marching by way of Emmaus, and the tenth by way of Jericho. Over and above these there were the auxiliaries of the kings, and many others from the province of Syria. And to fill the place of those whom Vespasian had chosen from the legions and sent on to Rome, there came two thousand men of the army of Alexandria and three thousand of the garrison that is on the river Euphrates. This was the army of Titus, and he had for chief counsellor, Tiberius Alexander, who aforetime had been Governor of Egypt.

This was the order of march with the army of Titus. First the auxiliaries from the kings; after these the pioneers; then the baggage of the captains with a guard; then Titus himself with his spearmen. After these the artillery; and after them the legions, marching six men abreast; then the slaves with the baggage; and last of all the mercenaries. And Titus pitched his camp in the Valley of Thorns, which is distant thirty furlongs from the City.

Then Titus took with him six hundred horsemen, and went forth to spy out the strength of the City. Also he had hopes that it might submit itself to him without a siege. For he had heard, as indeed was true, that the people were ill- disposed to the rebels, and would fain be at peace. And when he came near to the City by the way that slopes down to the walls, he saw no man, and the gates were shut. But when he approached the tower that is called Psephina, suddenly there burst forth from one of the gates a great multitude of men, and brake the array of the horsemen in twain, so that Titus with a few others was cut off from the rest. And indeed he could not go, forward, for the ground was broken with trenches, and divided with hedges and such like even up to the wall; and to go back was perilous, so great was the multitude of the enemy. Nor did the horsemen know how it was with him, but fled, thinking that he was with them. But he cried out to his companions that they should follow him, and drave right at the enemy to break through them. Then indeed might be seen the providence of God; for though javelins without number were cast at him, and he had neither helmet nor breastplate, for he had gone forth to spy and not to fight, yet did none wound him; but he let drive with his sword at them who stood near, and overthrew others with his horse. Then the Jews shouted aloud to see the courage of the man; and though they ceased not to encourage each other to assail him, yet for all that they gave place when he came near. And the other horsemen followed close behind him, seeing that thus only could they be saved. And in the end two only were taken and slain, but Titus and the others came back safe to his company. Neverthe-less, the Jews were much lifted up in hope by this matter, and thought that it was a fair beginning of great good fortune to come.

That night came the fifth legion by way of Emmaus. And the next day Titus went to a certain place called Scopus (which is by interpre-tation the "Outlook "), from which the City and the Temple could easily be seen; and it lieth on the north side of the City. Here he pitched a camp for two legions at seven furlongs from the City; and another for the fifth legion three furlongs behind. After this came the tenth legion by way of Jericho; to this it was commanded that it should pitch its camp on a hill called the Mount of Olives. This is distant six furlongs from the City, being divided from it by a deep valley, which is called the Valley of Cedron.

But when the three captains from within saw what was done, that the Romans were preparing to pitch three camps against the City, they began to take counsel among themselves. "Why," they said, "do we suffer the enemy to build these great works and we sit still, and use not our arms, as though these things concerned us not? We are bold enough against each other; but from our strife the Romans will gain this advantage, that they will take the City without loss." Then joining their bands together, and making a great shout, they rushed out upon the tenth legion, the same that was making its camp upon the Mount of Olives. Now the soldiers were busy about the work of entrenching, and had for the most part laid aside their arms; for they thought not that the Jews would dare to sally forth upon them, being also, they supposed, too much at variance among themselves for any such enterprise. Being therefore surprised, some fled, and others seeking to take up their arms were slain. And all the while the number of the Jews waxed greater and greater; and the Romans being used to fight in set array, were much perplexed by the suddenness and confusion of this onslaught. Wherefore though they stood their ground for a while, they were at the last driven out of the camp; and they had been in great peril of perishing altogether, but that Titus, seeing in what strait they were, came with certain chosen men, and fell upon the Jews, slaying many of them and driving them back into the valley of Cedron. And indeed as they were driven down the further slope of the valley they suffered much damage; but being come to the nearer side they gathered themselves together, and stood their ground against the Romans, having the river-bed in their midst. After this Titus bade his men fall back to the upper part of the hill, that they might finish the fortifying of the camp. But when the Jews perceived that he sent his men back, they took this for fear; and when the watcher whom they had set upon the wall gave the signal?and this he did by shaking his cloak?they ran forward, with others newly come from the City, and that with such swiftness that they seemed like to wild beasts. Nor could the legion sustain their attack, but the ranks were broken as though by the stones that are cast by artillery. Then was Titus left standing with a very few others; and though these would fain have him give way, for "it was not the part of a general," they said, "to fight as though he were but a soldier," yet he hearkened not to them, but stood his ground against the Jews as they ran up the hill, smiting them in the face, and slaying many, and driving them down the slope. But when they that were fortifying the camp saw that their fellows on the lower part of the hill gave way, they also fled, and the whole legion was scattered. But after a while certain soldiers perceived that Titus yet stood in the midst of the battle, and being in great fear of what might befall him, made this thing known to the others. Wherefore for very shame's sake they stayed their flight, reproaching each other that they had deserted their captain, and rushed with all their might upon the Jews, and drave them down the hill into the valley. And the Jews gave place, but ceased not nevertheless to fight. Then again Titus sent back the legion to finish the fortifying of the camp; and keeping with him those whom he had with him at the first, kept back the enemy.

After a few days there arose fresh strife in the City. It was now the Feast of the Passover; and Eleazar, the son of Simon, and his companions, opened the gates of the Temple, that such of the people as would worship might go in. Then John of Gischala took certain of his own company, choosing such as were not known to the Zealots, and commanded that they should hide their swords under their garments, and so go into the Temple. And many of these men had not been duly purified. When, therefore, they had been admitted, they threw aside their cloaks, so that it could be seen that they were armed. Then the Zealots left guarding the gates and leapt down from the battlements, hiding themselves in the passages that are under the Temple. But the people, not knowing what was about to be done, were gathered together round about the altar; and many of these were wounded and slain, for if any of the armed men had a grudge against any he used the occasion to satisfy it. Thus did the innocent suffer, but the guilty escaped; for John made a covenant with the Zealots that had fled into the passages under the Temple, saving them alive if they would serve him thenceforth. And he appointed Eleazar to be one of his captains. So now there were not three parties but two in Jerusalem, of whom John possessed the Temple and the Upper City; and Simon, the son of Gioras, the Lower City.

Titus was now purposed to bring his camps nearer to the City. And first he gave commandment that the whole space up to the walls should be made plain, and every hollow filled up, and every fruitful tree cut down. In the doing of this he suffered some loss, for the Jews drew certain of his men into an ambush, leading them within a stone's cast of the tower upon the wall. And this they did by a pretence of strife among themselves, for a company came without the walls, making as if they had been driven out by their fellows from within. But when the Romans followed, the whole army of the Jews ran forth from the gates and slew not a few. After this Titus, seeing that the whole space had been made plain according to his commandment, because he would move the baggage and the beasts of burden without damage, set the best of his soldiers in array from the northernmost point of the City to the westernmost. In the front he set the foot- soldiers, standing seven deep; and behind were the horsemen, in three companies, and in the midst were the archers. So all the baggage and the mixed multitude of the army passed safely behind the line; for the Jews could not break through them. Then were the camps pitched nearer to the City, being distant from it two furlongs only, of which camps one was at the corner of the wall which looketh to the south and to the west, and another was set at the tower which is called Hippicos, being also two furlongs from the City. As to the tenth legion it still abode in the Mount of Olives, which lieth to the east of the City.

8

OF THE WALLS OF JERUSALEM

THE City of Jerusalem had three walls, save only where it was defended by valleys that no man could pass; there indeed it had one only. The first wall compassed the New City; the beginning of it was at the Tower Hippicos, and the ending at the valley of Cedron. This King Agrippa built, for before his days the New City was without defence. But fearing the Emperor?in those days Claudius Cæsar was Emperor?lest he should be suspected of rebellion, he did not finish it according to his purpose. And indeed, if it had been so finished, it had been such that no man could have taken it. For the stones whereof it was built, being twenty cubits long, and ten cubits broad, could not easily be undermined or shaken with the battering rams. The height of it, when King Agrippa left building, was ten cubits only; but the Jews afterwards raised it to twenty cubits, adding thereto battlements and pinnacles, so that the measure of the whole was twenty-and-five cubits. The third wall, which is also the old wall, being the wall of the City of Sion, had its beginning in that corner of the Temple which looked to the north-west, and passed thence to the Tower Hippicos, and from the tower compassed the Upper City, along the valley of Hinnom, having its ending in the corner of the Temple that looked to the south- east. As for the second wall, it was built from the old wall, and had its ending at the Tower of Antony; and it compassed the Lower City.

On these walls there were towers, twenty cubits broad, and twenty in height, very strongly built and of beautiful stones, so that the Temple itself was not more fair. On every tower were chambers well furnished, and cisterns for rain. Of these towers the first wall had ninety, and the second fourteen, and the third sixty. Now the compass of the whole City was thirty-and-three furlongs.

The Tower of Antony stood at the corner of the Temple which looked to the north-west, being built upon a rock that was fifty cubits in height, and steep on all sides. It was the work of King Herod the Great, nor did he ever build anything more wonderful and magnificent. The face of the rock was cased with smooth stones; which thing was done both for the sake of ornament and also that no man might be able to ascend or descend thereby. Round the edge of the rock was a wall of three cubits, and within the wall the tower itself, having a height of forty cubits. Very wonderful was the tower both for greatness and for beauty, being divided into chambers of all kinds and fit for all uses; for it had halls, and cloisters, and baths, and courts that were convenient for the disposing of soldiers, so that it was as a city, for the number and variety of the things which it contained, and as a palace for its magnificence. On each corner also it had a tower, of which three were of the height of fifty cubits, and the fourth, being that which was near to the Temple, and looking to the south and the east, seventy-and-five cubits, so that a man could see from it the whole Temple. From this were steps to the cloisters that looked to the north and to the west, by which steps the soldiers that were on guard could go down when there might be occasion, for there were always soldiers in the tower; and these were especially diligent to watch the people on the feast days. For as the Temple was the fort of the City, so was the Tower of Antony the fort of the Temple.

As for the Temple, it was four-square, of a furlong each way. On two of its sides the rock served for a wall, and on two a wall was built;

nor was the height in any place less than three hundred cubits; and
certain of the stones that were used in the building were forty cubits
in length. Round about the Temple were double cloisters, built upon
pillars of white marble, very bright to look upon, and of the height of
twenty-and-five cubits. And the roof of the cloisters was of cedar, and
the whole circuit of these cloisters, together with the Tower of
Antony, was six furlongs. Within were open courts paved with all
manner of stones of divers colours. The outermost of these courts
was the Court of the Gentiles, having about it a wall of stone, very
cunningly made, and in this wall pillars whereon was written in
letters of Greek and Latin, "LET NO STRANGER ENTER THE HOLY
PLACE." (For the Inner Court was counted holy.) They that entered it
ascended by fourteen steps, and after the steps was a space of ten
cubits. Round about the Court was a wall of twenty-and-five cubits.
And all about this Court also were cloisters. On the west it had no
gate, but on the north four, and on the south four, and on the east
two. Of these gates the most wonderful by far was the Beautiful Gate,
being of the height of fifty cubits and of the breadth of forty cubits,
and made wholly of Corinthian brass. Within this Court was the
Holy Place, and before it a great porch, and in the porch, with twelve
steps going up thereto, a gate, but with no doors thereto, by which it
was signified that the heavens are not shut. And through this gate
could be seen the gate of the Holy Place, having over it the golden
vine, whereon were clusters of the bigness of a man's body. Over the
doors of this gate there hung a Babylonian curtain, of blue and yellow
and scarlet and purple; and by the blue was signified the air, and by
the yellow the earth, and by the scarlet fire, and by the purple the sea.
On this curtain also was wrought the likeness of the heavens. In this
Holy Place were the candlestick with seven branches (and the
number of the branches was seven because there are seven planets);
and the table of the shewbread, whereon were twelve loaves, because
the number of the months is twelve; and the altar of incense, with
incense of thirteen kinds, whereby it was signified that the earth is
the Lord's and the fulness thereof. Last of all was the Holy of Holies,
wherein there was nothing; nor was it lawful for any man to enter it

nor to look therein.

Without, the Temple was covered with great plates of gold, which glittered in the sun; and on the plates were great spikes, very sharp, that birds might not settle thereon.

9

THE SIEGE

WHEN Titus had ordered the camps for his army, he rode round the walls with chosen horsemen, looking for a place where he might assail them. And it befell that while he did this, one of his friends, Nicanor by name, was wounded by an arrow in the left shoulder. For he had gone near to the wall, and Josephus with him, thinking that being known to the people, he might incline their minds to peace. But Titus, when he knew this, made no more delay. For, dividing his army into three portions for the carrying on of the siege, he set slingers and archers on the banks which he had caused to be made, and behind the slingers his engines and artillery, to hinder such as would sally forth from the City against the siege-works. But the Jews on their part bestirred themselves. John, indeed, for fear of Simon, left not his place; but Simon set his machines of war upon the wall, both those which he had taken from Cestius, and those which he had got from the Tower of Antony. But his men for want of knowledge could not rightly use them; nevertheless, they somewhat troubled such as stood upon the banks. But the Romans, on the other hand, were defended by penthouses of wicker-work, and used their artillery to good purpose; the tenth legion having catapults and such-like machines of especial strength, so that they overthrew not only those that sallied from the gate, but also such as stood upon the walls, for they cast stones of a talent in weight, and cast them also two furlongs' space and more. At the first indeed the Jews were able to save themselves, because the stones were white and could be seen beforehand, by reason of their brightness. For men sat on the towers and watched, and cried out, when they saw the stone, IT COMETH, in the Hebrew tongue. Whereupon, they against whom it was sent would scatter themselves, and cast themselves on the ground, and the stone would fall harmless. But the Romans perceiving this, blackened the stones, so that they could not be seen beforehand. After this one stone would kill many men. For all this the Jews lost not heart, but day and night used both craft and valour to keep the Romans from the walls.

After this, Titus, perceiving that the battering rams could now be used against the wall?for the space between the banks and the wall had been measured by lead and line?commanded that they should be brought up; and at the same time he caused that his catapults should be brought nearer. Then the rams began to batter in three places. Which when they that were within perceived, seeing in what great peril they stood, they agreed to cease from their strife and make alliance against the enemy. Then Simon made proclamation that whosoever would might come forth from the Temple to the wall, and John, though he trusted him not, did not hinder any from going. Then did all the men of war join together, throwing lighted torches on to the machines, and casting darts without ceasing against them that served them; and some of the bolder sort sallied forth in companies, and tare down the penthouses with which the machines were covered. But Titus never ceased to help his men in their need, setting horsemen and archers on either side the machines to defend them, and driving back the darts thrown from the walls. Nevertheless the wall yielded not; only that the ram of the fifteenth legion brake down a corner of one of the towers; but the wall was not broken.

Then for a space the Jews ceased from their attacks; but when they saw that the Romans were somewhat scattered, the whole company of them sallied out together by the Tower Hippicos, seeking to set fire to the machines. Nay, so fiercely did they come on, that they reached even to the ramparts of the camp, nor could the Romans for all their good order stand against them. About the machines, indeed, the battle waxed very hot, and many were slain on both sides; and, indeed, the machines had been burnt, but for the valour of certain men of Alexandria, who bare themselves bravely beyond all expectation, standing fast till Titus came up with the most valiant of his horsemen. And Titus behaved himself most valiantly, slaying twelve men with his own hand. At the last all were driven back into the City, one man being taken captive, whom Titus commanded to be crucified for a terror to his countrymen.

This day, John, the captain of the Idumæans, was slain by an Arabian archer while he talked with a Roman of his acquaintance. Great lamentation was made for him, for he was a brave man and of a singular prudence.

Now, the Romans had built five towers, whereof the height was fifty cubits, on each bank a tower. By these the Jews were much harassed, for artillery of the lighter sort was set on them, together with slingers and archers. And they could not reach the top of the towers with arrows and the like by reason of their height; neither could they take them, nor overthrow them, so heavy were they (though, indeed, one fell, causing great fear among the Romans), nor burn them with fire, seeing that they were defended with iron. And if they sought to withdraw beyond the reach of the stones and darts, then they could not hinder the working of the rams, which, battering the wall without ceasing, began to make a breach. The biggest of these rams the Jews called THE CONQUEROR, because it conquered all things; and when this brake down the wall, and the Jews were wearied with fighting and watching, and considered also that there yet remained two walls, if this should be taken, they fled to the second wall. Then certain Romans climbing by the breach which The Conqueror had made, opened the gates. This happened on the fifteenth day from the beginning of the siege.

After this, Titus brought his camp within the first wall, and made preparation for attacking the second. And the Jews, on the other hand, were very zealous in defending it; and John defended the Tower of Antony and the north cloister of the Temple, and Simon defended what remained of the City. Many valiant deeds were done on both sides, of which may be mentioned those of Longinus, a Roman, and Castor, a Jew.

This Longinus was a knight, who, running forth from the host of the Romans, threw himself upon the Jews, breaking their line and slaying two of them. One he smote in the face, and the other he ran through as he fled, and both with the same spear. And when he had done this he came back to his friends unhurt.

As for Castor, he came forth, while the rams were battering the middle tower of the north wall, and stretching out his hands to Titus begged for grace. And Titus, believing him, for he hoped that the Jews were now weary of the siege, commanded that the rams should cease from their battering, and that the archers should stay their shooting. And he bade Castor say what he would have. Then said Castor, that he would fain give himself up to the Romans. And five of his companions seemed to agree with him (for he had ten men with him), but five affirmed that they would never serve the Romans. But while they disputed the siege was stayed; and of this Castor had sent warning to Simon bidding him see to such things as were urgent, for that he would deceive the Romans. Then he made as if he would persuade the others to yield, but they, with much show of indignation, were ready to slay themselves. And it so chanced that Castor was wounded in the nose by an arrow; whereupon he held out the arrow to Titus and made complaint. Then Titus rebuked the archer and bade Josephus draw near and give his hand to the man. But Josephus would not, knowing that the man meant nothing honest, and suffered not his friends to approach. Nevertheless a certain Æneas, a deserter, came near, and Castor cast a great stone at him, which hurt not Æneas, indeed, for he saw it as it came, but wounded a soldier that stood by. And when Titus saw that there was treachery, he commanded that the rams should begin their battering again. Then Castor and his companions set fire to the tower?for it was now sorely shaken?and made as if they leapt into the fire, for they, appeared to the Romans so to do, but in truth they leapt into a secret way which was ready prepared for them.

In the space of five days from the taking of the first wall, Titus took the second also. And if indeed he had thrown down the greater part of it or had destroyed that part of the City which lay between the two walls, he had suffered no damage. But this he did not, hoping that the Jews, when they saw his moderation, would be the more inclined to yield themselves to him. Therefore he gave commandment that the prisoners should not be slain, nor the houses burnt; for he would gladly have preserved the City for himself, and the Temple for the City. But the men of war would not so much as endure a word concerning peace, but sallied forth from the lanes of the City and from the houses, and set on the Romans that were come within the wall. And because they were more in number, and also knew the place, they did them much damage; and though these stood firm?and indeed they could not flee by reason of the narrowness of the gates? they were in great straits, and this the more because the men in the towers had fled; and they had doubtless perished all of them but that Titus came to their help: who, setting archers at the lanes' ends, kept back the Jews till he had drawn all his soldiers outside of the wall.

The Jews took heart when they saw the Romans driven back, thinking that these would not dare to attack them again, and that their City should never be taken; for God blinded their eyes by reason of their sins, so that they thought not how that the Romans had a host many times greater than that which they had driven back, nor remembered that famine also was coming before them. For three days they fought steadfastly against the Romans, filling the breaches in the wall with their bodies; but after this they gave place, and fled within the third wall; and Titus, having taken possession of the second wall, cast down that part which looked to the north; as for the southern part, he set guards in the towers, and so addressed himself to the taking of the third wall.

10

THE SIEGE (CONTINUED)

NEVERTHELESS it seemed good to Titus to cease from the siege for awhile, that he might give to the Jews a place of repentance, if haply, seeing that the second wall was now taken and that their provision of food also was failing them, they might be inclined to surrender themselves and the City. To this same end he brought all his soldiers under review; who having taken the coverings from their arms and having clad themselves in their breastplates, marched before the walls; and the horsemen also led horses very splendidly arrayed; so that the whole space before the City glittered with gold and silver. And in the City the old wall and the northern part of the Temple and the houses were filled with spectators. Great was the fear of the Jews to behold so great a host and so well equipped; and many of the rebels would willingly have surrendered themselves. But the ringleaders would not; for knowing that they should suffer punishment for their misdeeds, they judged it far better to die in battle; nor did they care if the City should perish with them.

Four days were spent in the distributing to each legion of needful provision; and on the fifth day Titus divided his army into two parts, whereof one was to assail the Tower of Antony and the other the Third Wall (which was called also the Old Wall). But as he would fain have saved the City, he made yet another trial of the Jews, sending to them Josephus, who, standing in a place whence his words could be heard, being yet beyond a javelin throw from the walls, exhorted and entreated them in many words. "Can ye hope;" he said, "two walls having been taken, that the third, which is weaker than they, will hold out? And why do ye disdain the Romans as masters, to whom God hath manifestly given the dominion of the whole world? And now indeed they are willing to have mercy on you, but if ye resist, then of a truth when they shall have taken the City they will spare no one; and that they must needs take it is manifest, seeing that, if their arms prevail not, yet ye must be subdued by hunger."

And when they laughed him to scorn, and some cast javelins at him, he recounted how God had dealt with the nation in past time; giving them many and great deliverances, but these only if they were obedient to His word; and how Zedekiah, king of Judah, when he fought with the Chaldeans against the word of Jeremiah the prophet, was led into captivity, and the City and the Temple of God were destroyed. And that God was with the Romans was manifest, he said, both from many other things and because Siloam and all other springs that are without the City, having been dried up before when the Jews had them in possession, now gave abundance of water. With these and many other like words, Josephus besought the people that they would make agreement with the Romans.

John and Simon, and they that followed after them, paid no heed to these words; but many of the people were moved thereby to escape to the Romans; of whom some sold their goods, and some swallowed their most precious things. Titus permitted them to go whithersoever they would; but the chiefs of the rebels were very fierce against all who would fly from the City, and slew those whom they so much as suspected of this purpose.

And now the famine grew more and more grievous every day. Of public stores there was nothing; but the soldiers would enter the houses to search for food; which if they found they would scourge them that dwelt there as having sought to conceal it, and if they found nought, then they would torture them the more cruelly as if they would discover it. Indeed they judged from men's look whether or no they had food; and such as were in good case they judged to have abundance, and such as were wasted to have nothing. Many sold their goods for a peck of wheat, or if they were poor, even of barley. This they would carry into the inner part of their dwelling, and for stress of hunger would eat the corn unground. And they took no heed of shame or natural affection; but wives would snatch the food from their husbands, and children from their parents, aye, and mothers from their babes. Nor were they suffered to devour in peace what they got in this evil fashion; but if the soldiers saw anywhere a house shut up they concluded that food was hidden therein, and entering in spared neither old nor young, woman or child, compelling them by cruelties and torments to deliver up all that they possessed. And this they did, not under stress of hunger, but that they might store up for themselves food for many days. And if any crept out secretly at night without the walls to gather herbs of the field, or such- like things, on these they would lay hands as they came back, and take from them all that they had found; not suffering them, for all their entreaties, to keep ought for themselves. But when Titus perceived that the number of them that came out of the City seeking for food daily increased, he commanded that such as were taken so doing should be crucified before the walls. For to let them go free he judged to be dangerous; nor was he willing to keep a great multitude of captives. And, besides, he had hopes that the sight of them would incline them that were within the City to surrender themselves. But as they paid no heed to it, he bade the soldiers proceed with the siege-works.

Meanwhile there came into the camp of the Romans a certain Antiochus Epiphanes, son to the King of Commagene, than whom there was in those days no tributary of the Empire more prosperous. This young man had with him a company of noble youths, whom he called his Macedonians, being clad and armed in the fashion of that nation. And the young man, who was of great courage and strength, wondered, he said, that the Romans delayed to attack the wall. Which when Titus heard, he laughed, and said, "Ye can have your share;" whereupon the young man, with his comrades, as they were, made an attack upon the wall.

But though Antiochus himself was not hurt, yet all the youths that were with him, save a very few only, were wounded or slain; for they persevered to the last, remembering how they had boasted of what they could do.

And now there had been raised four banks against the wall of the City, four legions having laboured at them for the space of seventeen days. But John and his men had undermined the whole space that lay between the Tower of Antony and the banks, and having stored therein pitch and sulphur and such-like things, set fire to them, so that the timbers whereupon the earth was supported being burnt through, all the works fell in; not without great dismay and discouragement to the Romans.

Two days after this, Simon made, upon his part, an attack upon the battering rams. Certain men, being the bravest of all his company, taking torches in their hands, set fire to the rams, nor would they suffer themselves to be driven back by all the swords and darts of the Romans till the engines began to burn. And when the soldiers ran together to quench the fire, the Jews upon the wall hindered them with darts, and others ran forth from the gates and fought with them. The Romans, indeed, sought to carry away the rams, though the coverings were consumed, but the Jews would not loose their hold, for all that the iron was now heated red-hot. And now the Romans, having no hope that they could save the artillery, fell back into the camp; whither also the Jews pursued them, for multitudes came forth from the City continually to help them, so that they joined battle even with them that guarded the fortifications of the camp. Now, the Romans have a law whereby they punish with death any man that deserteth his post, wherefore the guards fought the more steadfastly.

Yet for all this could they not turn back the Jews, so fiercely did they come on. Yea, even when Titus himself came up with a company of soldiers, they turned upon him and fought as men who had no care for their lives; and at last, having caused great damage and loss to the Romans, they returned to the City.

11

THE TAKING OF THE CITY

TITUS held a consultation with his captains what it were best to do. Some that were of a fierce temper said that it would be well to make an instant assault on the wall with the whole army, for the Jews, they said, have hitherto fought with a part only, nor will they be able to stand up against the whole, but will be overwhelmed by the javelins alone. But others said that they should raise new banks against the wall. And others again that they should blockade the City, so that none should go out or in, and so leave the people to perish with hunger. To Titus himself it seemed a base thing that so great an army should sit doing nothing; yet he judged it an idle thing to fight with men that cared nothing for their lives. And as for blockading the City, this, he thought, would be a very difficult thing, for that the Jews would find out some secret ways of coming out and going in, and that there was danger lest the glory of their enterprise should be diminished, if the City should thus have power to hold out for some long time. He judged, therefore, that it would be best to surround the whole City with a wall, by which means their work would be both safely and speedily accomplished.

This therefore was done; and the soldiers worked with such diligence and zeal, that the wall was built in the space of three days. It was thirty-and-nine furlongs in length, and on the outer side thereof there stood thirteen forts. And that it might be the more diligently guarded, Titus himself kept the first watch, and Alexander, that had been Governor of Egypt, the second, and the captains of the legions the third.

But in the City, now that all power and hope of going forth had been taken away, the famine grew daily more grievous, and many perished of hunger, gazing earnestly on the Temple; and their dead bodies lay in the houses and in the streets, for there was no man to bury them. At the first, indeed, they buried the dead at the charge of the treasury, but afterwards, the number increasing, they cast them over the heights into the valleys and ravines. But when Titus, riding about the City, saw this sight, for it was a very grievous thing to behold, and there came also a horrible stench from the corpses, he lifted up his hands, and called God to witness that this was not of his doing. And because he had compassion on the people, and would save some of them, at the least, from perishing with hunger, he set his army again to siege-works, casting up banks against the Tower of Antony, which mounds were larger by far than had been cast up at the first; and because all the trees in the neighbourhood of the City had been cut down, the soldiers fetched the timber from the distance of ninety furlongs and more.

Meanwhile, in the City, the high priest Matthias was put to death, together with his sons; being accused of a purpose to betray the City to the Romans. And when the old man besought that he might be slain the first, they would not hearken to him, but slew his sons before his eyes, and himself last of all. And this they did in the sight of the Romans.

Also, when a certain Judas, who was of the captains of Simon, repenting him of all this wickedness, made a plot with ten others to deliver up the Temple to the Romans, Simon, having discovered the matter, slew all of them and cast their bodies down from the wall.

About this time Josephus, as he went about the wall (for he ceased not to persuade his countrymen that they should yield them-selves to the Romans), was smitten on the head with a stone, and fell senseless to the ground. And the Jews sallied forth to lay hands upon him, and would doubtless have carried him into the City, but that Titus sent certain soldiers to his help.

Of the Jews many cast themselves down from the wall, being driven thereto by hunger: and others, making as if they would go forth to battle, fled to the Romans. Of these, many perished most miserably; for some eating and drinking without stint after long fasting, so died; and others were slain by Arabians and Syrians in the camp. For it had been noised abroad that many of them that escaped from the city had swallowed gold?of which indeed there was great plenty?and the Arabians and Syrians slew many for the sake of what they might find in their bodies. But when Titus heard of these doings he was very wroth, and but for the multitude of the guilty, would have surrounded them with horsemen and cut them in pieces. But because they were so many, he called together the captains of the auxiliaries and of the legions also (for certain of the Romans themselves were accused of the same crime), and affirmed that he would put to death any who should thereafter be discovered so doing. Nevertheless this greed of gain prevailed over the fear of death, and many of them that escaped from the City were still slain in this fashion.

And now John, not content with the evil that he had done already, began to commit sacrilege. For he took of the gifts and offerings of the Temple, bowls and dishes and tables (and among these the pitchers which Augustus the Emperor and Livia his wife had offered), and melted them for the coining of money. Also he took the sacred wine and oil which should be kept for the use of the priests only, and distributed them to his soldiers, who feared not to drink of the wine and anoint themselves with the oil. Verily it is to be believed that if the Romans had delayed to destroy these wicked men, the earth had opened her mouth for them, or they had been swept away by a flood, or had perished by the fire of Sodom.

And now the Romans had finished their siege-works, for which indeed they had consumed all the trees that were within ninety furlongs of the City; nor if these should be destroyed did they know how they should make others. For which reason they regarded them not without fear; and the Jews also seeing their bigness, and how near they were to the wall, were greatly terrified. And though John and his followers, issuing forth from the Temple, sought to set fire to them, they harmed them not at all; nor indeed did they bear themselves as valiantly as they had been wont to do. And on the other hand, the Romans kept more steadfastly to their places than before, standing in such close array that the fire could not be brought near to the machines; so that after no long conflict the Jews fell back into the City. Whereupon the Romans brought the rams up to the wall, nor were they hindered by the stones and darts and such- like things that they who stood upon the Tower of Antony poured down upon them; but they closed their shields over their heads, and under cover of these brake away the foundations of the work with their hands and with levers, so that at nightfall they had with much labour moved from their places four great stones.

But during the night the wall of a sudden fell down, for the ground beneath it had been mined; yet the work was not finished, for John had built another wall behind the former one. Only this, it seemed, could be more easily taken than the first one, the ruins whereof were a help to them that would attack; also being newly built it had not the strength of the old wall. For all this none among the Romans dared to approach it. But when Titus had exhorted his soldiers, promising rewards to them that should venture on this work and live, and fame without end to such as should fall in the doing of it, a certain Sabinus, who was of the auxiliaries, a Syrian by nation, came forth and said, "O Cæsar, willingly do I offer myself for this work, and will be the first to climb the wall." And indeed he was a man of great strength and courage, though to look upon him he scarcely seemed fit for a soldier, for he was small and slight of stature. Then, having drawn his sword, and holding his shield over his head with his left hand, he ran forward to the wall; and there followed him eleven others and no more. And though the guards on the wall cast stones and javelins without number against him, striking down with them some of the eleven, yet him they harmed not till he had climbed on to the top of the wall, for the Jews were astonished at his courage, and fled before him, thinking also that more must needs be following him. But when he had well-nigh accomplished his undertaking there befell him (as indeed often happens in such enterprises) a very ill chance, for he stumbled upon a stone and fell with a great crash. Which when the Jews perceived, seeing him lie on the top of the wall alone, they turned upon him; and though he defended himself and wounded many of the enemies, yet at last his strength failed him; and indeed he was buried under a multitude of spears even before he died. Of the eleven three were slain, and the rest carried back to the camp grievously wounded.

But two days afterwards, twenty of them that guarded the banks, taking with them a standard-bearer of the fifth legion, and two horsemen, and a trumpeter, at the ninth hour of the night approached silently to the Tower of Antony, and finding the sentinels asleep, slew them, and so mounted on the wall; which when they had done, they bade the trumpeter sound on his trumpet; and the guards of the wall, hearing the trumpet, fled, judging that it would not have sounded had not many been present, and Titus, on the other hand, commanded the soldiers to arm themselves with all haste; and himself came with a chosen company of men. Thus did the Romans take possession of the Tower of Antony; but when the Romans pressed on and would have taken the Temple also, John and Simon, joining their forces together, drave them back into the Tower. Thus for ten hours, even from the ninth hour of the night until the seventh hour of the day, they fought; and many were slain on both sides. Among these there was none more worthy to be remembered than Julianus, a centurion, a man of a singular strength and courage, who, when he perceived that the Romans gave place to the Jews (for he was standing by Titus in the Tower), leapt forward, and with his own hand only put the Jews to flight, and drave them before him so far as to the corner of the Inner Court, slaying many, to the great admiration of Cæsar and terror of the enemy. But here his fate overtook him; for having in his shoes many and sharp nails, as soldiers are wont to have, he slipped on the polished pavement of the Temple and so fell. Thereupon the Jews turned upon him; nor could he raise himself from the ground for the multitude of them that assailed him; and so after wounding many he perished, Cæsar greatly grieving that so brave a man should be slain, and that where none could give him any help. So the Romans abode for awhile in the Tower of Antony.

But Titus judged it best that the Tower should be laid even with the ground, so that the army might the more easily approach to the Temple. Yet he would try the Jews once more if they would yield themselves, for he had heard that the daily sacrifice had ceased for the want of men to offer it. Therefore he sent Josephus again to John and his fellows; who, standing where he could be heard by all the people, spake to them in the Hebrew tongue, that they might have pity on their country and on the Temple of God. And when John answered that he feared not what might happen, for that the City was the City of God, Josephus reproached him with all that he had done against the Temple, saying, nevertheless, that he had yet a place of repentance if he would yield himself. John, indeed, would not hearken to these words, but many of the nobles hearkened, and delivered themselves to Titus, who dealt kindly with them. But the Jews gave out that they had been slain, lest others should do likewise; which when Titus heard, he bade them show themselves in the sight of all the people, who, when they saw them, were the more inclined to come over to the Romans. After this, Titus spake to John and his fellows, saying, "Dost thou not know that we have always held this Temple sacred, which thou hast defiled with slaughter, setting certain boundaries, which if any stranger over-passed it was lawful for you to put him to death? And now I swear to you by the gods of my country that if ye will take another place for your fighting, no Roman shall come "near to the Temple." All this he said, using Josephus for his interpreter.

But the rebels, thinking that he spake this for fear, were confirmed in their folly. Therefore Titus delayed no longer to attack the Temple. And because there was not space for all his army, he chose thirty out of every company, and set a tribune over every thousand, and appointed Cerealis to be captain of all. To these he gave commandment that they should attack the guards of the Temple at the ninth hour of the night. And he would have gone with them himself, but his friends hindered him, saying that he would serve them better if he stood by the Tower of Antony, and ordered the battle, and that the soldiers also would fight the better, as knowing that they were under the eyes of Cæsar. Therefore he sat in a watch tower to see what should happen.

Then there was fought a very fierce battle. For the Romans found not the guards sleeping as they had hoped; but these raised the alarm, and the whole multitude came to their help. And each knew their friends indeed by their speech, but could not see them for the darkness, which indeed caused fear to some and madness to others, so that they smote all whom they approached, without discrimination. But the Romans, seeing that they advanced in order, and had watchwords, were less troubled by the darkness than were the Jews. For the most part the battle was fought by both as they stood, for neither had space either for flying or for pursuing. And they that stood by the Tower shouted to their fellows, if they saw them prevail, that they should go yet further, and bade them be of good heart, if they saw them beaten back. They fought from the ninth hour of the night till the fifth hour of the day, and neither had the advantage.

After this, the Tower of Antony having been now destroyed, the legion made a broad way of approach to the Temple, and began to cast up banks against it, surrounding it on the north side, and on the east, and on the west.

The next day after the finishing of this way, many of the Jews, being sore pressed by hunger, attacked the garrison of the Romans that was on the Mount of Olives, about the eleventh hour of the day, hoping to find them taking their rest. But the Romans, being aware beforehand of their coming, met them and hindered them from breaking through the wall. And though the Jews fought fiercely as men who despaired of life, yet they gained nothing, but were driven back to the City. And here a certain Pedanius, a horseman, made himself a great name; for he caught up a young man of the enemy as he fled, with marvellous strength of arm and skill of horsemanship, and carried him to Titus.

And now the Jews, seeing that the war daily came nearer and nearer even to the Temple, did as one that cuts off a diseased limb that he may save the rest of his body; for they set fire to the cloister which was between the Temple and the Tower of Antony, to the length of twenty cubits; part also the Romans burned, so that the whole space between the Temple and the Tower was now empty.

About these days a certain Jonathan came out of the City and called to the Romans to send a man to fight with him. And as no man answered he began to scoff at them for their fear, till a certain Pudens, thinking that he should easily prevail (for the Jew was short and weak to look upon), came forth. And indeed he had the better in the fight, but stumbled by chance, and so was slain by Jonathan. Then the Jew, putting his foot on the dead body, shook his sword in one hand and his shield in the other, boasting of his deed, till a certain Priscus, a centurion, shot him through with an arrow.

12

THE TAKING OF THE CITY

T HE Jews that were in the Temple caused no small loss to the Romans by this device. Having filled the space that was between the beams and the roof of the cloister that stood westward of the Temple with wood and sulphur and bitumen, they fell back as though they were wearied of defending. Whereupon many of the Romans set ladders against it and climbed on to the top; but the wiser sort remained in their place. So soon then as the cloister was covered with them that had climbed on to it, the Jews put fire underneath, so that in a very short space the flames surrounded it on every side. Then some leapt down among their friends, and some among the enemy, breaking their limbs for the most part in the fall; and many were destroyed by the fire; and some slew themselves with. their swords, judging it better so to die. Among these last was a certain Longus, to whom the Jews promised his life if he would yield himself to them. But his brother Cornelius exhorted him not so to disgrace his name and country; whereupon the young man lifted up his sword in the sight of both armies and slew himself. Of those who were cut off by the fire, one Artorius saved his life by craft. He called with a loud voice to a certain fellow-soldier, Lucius by name, saying, "I will leave thee all my goods if thou wilt come hither and receive me when I fall." So the man came, and Artorius leaping down upon him was saved, but Lucius being dashed upon the pavement died forthwith. The western cloister being now burnt the Romans also set fire to that which stood on the north of the Temple.

In these days the famine increased, and the inhabitants of the City suffered such things by reason of it as it is not possible to tell. For in every household if there was to be seen so much as the shadow of food, there was war, men contending with them that were dearest to them. And now even the soldiers were hard pressed by hunger, and ran about through the City as greedy dogs, and scarcely knew for weakness whither they went. And necessity compelled them to devour all manner of things, so that they would gather for themselves even such as the vilest of brute beasts use not; they eat also their girdles and sandals, and tearing the leather thongs from their shields they rent them with their teeth. And some devoured morsels of dried grass; and others gathered leaves of trees; these indeed were sold for a great weight of silver.

But what men did in the fury of their hunger with such things as these is of small account; for now there must be related such a deed as was never told of the Greeks, or of the Romans, or of any tribe of the barbarians; a most horrible thing in truth and scarcely to be believed.

There was a certain woman of the region that lieth eastward of Jordan, and her name was Mary, the daughter of Eleazar, of Bethezob, which is by interpretation the "house of hyssop." She was of a noble house and wealthy, and had taken refuge in the City. But the men of war had robbed her of all the possessions which she had brought with her from beyond Jordan. This had stirred her up to great anger, and she reproached the men daily with all manner of hard words and revilings; but when no man would slay her either for anger or for pity, and she was grievously tormented by hunger, she did a horrible deed and contrary to nature, for she caught up the sucking child that she had, and roasted his flesh, and having eaten the half of it herself put by that which was left. And in a short space of time came the men of war, for they smelt the savour of the food, and threatened that they would slay her forthwith, if she would not bring forth that which she had prepared. And the woman said, "I have kept a goodly portion for you," and uncovered that which remained of her son. And when the men stood astonished, she cried, "Eat ye, even as I have eaten. Why should ye be softer than a woman or more merciful than a mother? But if perchance ye have a scruple, and will not eat of my sacrifice, then as I have eaten the half, so may ye leave me that which remains." And the men departed trembling. This thing was noised abroad throughout the City, and all who heard it said that they were happy indeed who had died before that they had seen or heard such things.

But when this came to the ears of Titus, he protested that this was not of his doing, for that he had offered to the Jews peace, and to be governed according to their own laws, and pardon for all that had been done; but that they, having refused these things, deserved that such dreadful things should come upon them. At the same time he was now certain in himself that there was no more hope that the Jews would come to a sound mind so as to yield themselves to him.

On the eighth day of the month of August, the rams began to batter the western gate of the Inner Court; but when they had battered for six days and had done nothing, neither could the stones be moved by levers and the like, Titus commanded the soldiers that they should get to the cloisters and climb on to them. But this also they could not accomplish, for many were slain to no purpose, and certain standards also were taken. Then Titus, being unwilling that his soldiers should suffer this loss any more, commanded that they should set fire to the gates. When this had been done, the silver melting, the fire made its way to the wood and spread quickly to the cloisters round about; nor did the Jews seek to quench it, for they were as men that had lost all hope. All that day and night therefore the fire burned; and on the morrow Titus, having given commandment to some of the soldiers that they should extinguish the fire and clear the way to the Temple, called a council of his chief captains. Some thought that the Temple should he destroyed, for that the Jews would never cease to rebel so long as they should have this refuge whereunto they could fly. Others thought that the Temple might be spared, if only the Jews would leave it, for that now it was not a temple but a fort. But Titus said, "That even it, the Jews should make war from the Temple, yet would he spare it, for that he would not avenge on that which had no life the wickedness of many and that it would be a shame to the Roman people if that should be destroyed which was the glory of the whole world."

That day the Jews rested and did nothing; but on the morrow they took courage and issued forth from the eastern gate against them that kept the Outer Court. This they did about the second hour of the day. And doubtless they had overcome them, being more in number, only Titus, seeing what had befallen from the Tower of Antony, came to the help of the Romans with certain horsemen. The Jews could not stand before him, but were forced to flee; yet when the Romans retreated they turned again to the attack; but at the last, about the fifth hour of the day, were driven back into the Inner Court of the Temple.

Then Titus, being resolved that on the morrow he would attack the Temple with all his might, went back to the Tower of Antony. But indeed the day was come when it was appointed that it should perish, being the self-same day on which the former Temple had been burnt by the King of Babylon. But now the beginning of the destruction was from the Jews themselves; for, when Titus had departed, these, having rested awhile, set again upon the Romans in the Outer Court, who were seeking to quench the burning of the cloisters. These, putting the Jews to flight, came in their pursuit as far as the Inner Court. Whereupon a certain soldier, lifting himself on the shoulders of a comrade, cast a torch which he had caught up from the burning, through a door in the wall, from which access was had to the chambers that were about the Temple on the north side. This he did without any commandment given, but, as it would seem, by a certain Divine inspiration. And when the Jews saw the fire, for it rose up forthwith, they set up a great cry, and ran to help, for they did not care to live now that the place which they had defended was ready to perish.

Then one ran to tell Titus, who lay asleep in his tent. And forthwith he ran with all speed to the Temple, if he might hinder the burning, the captains following him and a great multitude of men with them. But though he cried to the soldiers, and signed also with his hand that they should quench the burning, it profited nothing, for they could neither see nor hear him for the noise and tumult. And as for the multitude that followed, they took no heed of anything, but rushed with all speed into the Temple, trampling one another down in the narrow gateways, and stumbling on the ruins, so that many perished along with the enemy. And the commands of Titus they heard not, or made as if they heard not, but cast firebrands on to that which was not yet burning, and slaughtered multitudes of the people, so that the dead bodies were piled up against the altar, and the blood flowed down the steps of the Temple.

Then Titus, seeing that he could not stay the fury of the soldiers, and that the fire increased continually, entered with his captains into the Holy Place. Yet, seeing how beautiful it was and richly adorned, beyond all report that had gone forth of its beauty and riches, and that the fire had not yet touched it, but consumed the outer chambers, he sought yet once more to save it, crying out to the soldiers that they should quench the fire, and to Liberalis, the centurion of his bodyguard, to lay hands on such as were disobedient. But wrath and hatred of the enemy, and the desire of plunder, prevailed over their reverence for Cæsar. And at last a certain soldier, not being seen, for the place was dark, thrust a lighted torch between the hinges of the door; whereupon the flame rose up in a moment, and Titus and his captains were driven perforce out of the place. Thus did the Temple perish. And from the building of the First Temple, by Solomon, were one-thousand-one-hundred-and-thirty years and seven months and fifteen days, and from the building of the Second Temple, in the days of Cyrus the Persian, six-hundred-and-thirty-nine years and forty-five days.

And while the Temple was burning, the soldiers ceased not to slay all whom they met; nor had they pity for youth, or reverence for old age, but put both old and young, people and priests, to the sword. And there went up a great and terrible clamour, the soldiers shouting aloud for joy, and the Jews crying out as they saw themselves surrounded with fire and sword, and the people bewailing the Temple, for even they who could scarce speak for the weakness of hunger, when they saw the burning of the Holy Place brake forth with loud lamentations. As for the Temple, and the hill whereon it stood, the ground could not be seen for dead bodies; and the soldiers trampled on heaps of corpses as they pursued them that fled. As for the rebels, the greater part of them brake through the ranks of the Romans into the Outer Court, and so escaped into the Upper City. Some of the priests used the spits of the service of the Temple and the seats, which were of lead, for missiles which they might cast against the Romans; and two of them, when they might have yielded themselves to Titus, or fled with their companions, threw themselves into the fire, and so perished.

The Romans, indeed, thinking that the Temple being burnt, it profited nothing to save that which was left, set fire to all the buildings that were round about it, so that two only of the gates were left, and these also they afterwards destroyed. The treasury also was burnt, in which there was treasure that could not be counted, and garments without number, and ornaments, and, indeed, all the riches of the nation of the Jews. And now there remained one cloister of the Outer Court, in which were gathered many women and children, and a mixed multitude of men, six thousand in all. And to this, before Titus gave any commandment in the matter, the soldiers in their fury set fire; and these all perished. Now the cause why they were gathered together in the cloister was this. A certain false prophet had said, "Hear the word of the Lord. Go ye up into the Temple, and the Lord shall give you there signs of deliverance." And, indeed, the seditious suborned many false prophets to speak to the people, saying that the Lord would help them, that they might not go over to the Romans.

Yet were there many manifest signs and portents by which the desolation to come was signified; but they would not believe or understand. For they were as men smitten with madness, and blinded both in eyes and heart; and heeded not the tokens of God. For, first of all, there stood over the City a star that had the form of a sword, and a comet that ceased not to burn for the space of a whole year. Also before the beginning of the war, when the people were assembled for the Passover, on the eighth day of the month Nisan, at the ninth hour of the night, there shone round about the Temple and the altar a light as great as the light of noonday; and this endured for the space of half-an-hour. This thing the unlearned took for a sign of good things to come; but the Scribes judged that it portended the evils which indeed came to pass afterwards. A heifer also in the same feast, when the priest was leading it to the altar for sacrifice, brought forth a lamb in the midst of the Temple. Also the door of the Holy Place, looking to the westward, being wholly of bronze, and of a very great weight, so that when it was shut in the evening, twenty men could scarce move it, and which had bolts of iron, and posts of stone in one piece, driven very deep into a threshold of stone, was found open of its own accord about the sixth hour of the night. Which thing the keepers of the Temple ran and told to the captain, and he, coming with others, was scarcely able to shut it. This also seemed to the ignorant and unlearned a very excellent sign, that God had opened to the people a gate of good things; but the learned thought that this rather was signified by it, that the Temple, having been safe heretofore, now opened its gates to the enemy, and that desolation was about to come upon it. Also on certain days after the festival there appeared a thing so marvellous as to be beyond belief, but that it was related by many that saw it with their own eyes. Before the setting of the sun there were seen chariots driven across the sky, and hosts of armed men setting themselves in order of battle, and surrounding cities. And on the day of Pentecost, when the priests entered the Temple at night to do after the manner of their office, they heard the sound as of many feet, and the voice as of a great multitude saying, LET US GO HENCE. But a thing yet more terrible than these is yet to he told. A certain Joshua, the son of Ananus, a countryman, and one of the common folks, four years before the beginning of the war, the City being at peace and abounding with all manner of stores, began of a sudden to cry out, "A voice from the east; a voice from the west; a voice from the four winds; a voice against Jerusalem, and against the

Temple; a voice against the bridegroom and the bride; a voice against the whole people." And he went about through the streets of the City crying these words both day and night. Then some of the chief of the people, taking it ill that he should say continually words of such evil meaning, laid hands upon him and scourged him. But he spake not one word for himself, nor made supplication to them that scourged him, but ceased not to cry out as before. After this, the rulers of the people, thinking that he spake by some power that was more than that of a man (and this indeed was so), brought him before the Roman governor. But though the governor caused him to he scourged, even to the laying bare of his bones, the man used neither entreaties nor tears. Only at every stroke he cried out as loud as he could with a very lamentable voice, "Woe to Jerusalem." And when Albinus asked him (for Albinus was governor in those days), "Who art thou, and whence didst thou come? and why sayest thou these things?" Joshua answered him not a word, but ceased not to make lamentation over the City, till Albinus, judging that he was mad, let him depart. And the man, until the beginning of the war, neither came into any house, nor spake to any man, but lamented in these words, "Woe to Jerusalem." Nor, though he was beaten daily, did he curse any man, nor did he bless any that gave him food, but his answer to all was in these words only. And he was most instant in crying them on feast days. And when he had done this for the space of seven years and five months (yet his voice was not hoarse, nor he himself weary), at the last, when his prophecy was now fulfilled, he ceased from his crying. For on a certain day, as he went about on the walls and cried, after his custom, "Woe to the City, and to the Temple, and to the people," of a sudden he added, "woe also to myself." And when he had said these words, a stone from one of the engines smote him that he died.

Whoever will note these things may know that God hath a care for men, and showeth them beforehand such things as concern their welfare, and that if they perish, they perish from their own madness and the evil of their own choosing. So there was a certain oracle: "The Temple and the City shall be taken when the shape of the Temple shall be four-square." And this, indeed, came to pass when the Tower of Antony was taken and destroyed. But the thing that more than all stirred the people up to war, was a certain saying that was found in their Scriptures, "In those days there shall go forth from this land one who shall be Lord of the whole world." These words they took to themselves, so that many even of the wiser sort were deceived by a false interpretation, nor did they know that it was signified thereby that Vespasian should he made Emperor.

13

THE END

W HEN the rebels had fled into the Upper City, the Temple and all the cloisters about it being now on fire, the Romans set their standards by the eastern gate, and did sacrifice, and saluted Titus as Emperor with a very great shouting. So much plunder had the soldiers from the spoiling of the Temple, that at this time a pound weight of gold was sold in Syria for half only of the price that it had before.

There were certain of the priests who had climbed on to the wall of the Temple and would not descend; and among these a boy who, being tormented with thirst, cried out to the Roman guards that they should reach him a hand that he might come down, for that he was dying from thirst. And when, having compassion on his youth, one of them reached to him his hand, he came down, and drank himself, and filled his pitcher with water, and having so done, fled back to his own people; nor could any of the guards overtake him. On the fifth day the priests, being now overcome with hunger, came down, and besought Titus that he would have compassion upon them; but he made answer to them that the day of mercy was now past, and commanded that they should be slain.

After this Simon and John, and they that were with them, seeing

that they were surrounded and had now no way of escape, said that
they would speak with Titus. And he, for that he was of a gentle
temper, and would gladly have saved the City, and being also
persuaded by his friends, said that he would hear them. Wherefore
he stood on the Terrace, that was on the western side of the Temple,
where there was a bridge between the Temple and the Upper City,
and spake with them, having first commanded the soldiers that they
keep their wrath within bounds, and should not shoot arrows against
them that stood on the other side of the bridge. And first he rebuked
them for their folly, in that they had thought to resist the Romans,
who had conquered all the nations of the world, as the Germans, for
all the greatness of their stature, and the Britons, for all that they had
the sea for a defence. Also he brought up against them, that, even
after he had begun to besiege the City, he had yet been willing to
make peace, and had besought them to have compassion on themselves, and on their countrymen, and on the Holy Place. "And now,"
he said, "that your Temple hath perished, are ye worthy to live? Yet
even now ye come not as suppliants to me, but stand in arms against
me, though your nation hath perished, and I have the mastery over
your City. Nevertheless, if ye will lay down your arms, and yield yourselves to me, I give you your lives." To this the rebels made answer,
"Thy hand we cannot take, for we have sworn a great oath that this
thing we will not do. But if thou wilt suffer us to go forth with our
wives and our children, we will depart into the desert, and leave this
City to thee." At which words the wrath of Titus was greatly moved;
and he bade a herald proclaim that thenceforth he would spare no
man, but would deal with them after the custom of war. Then he
commanded the soldiers to spoil and burn all that remained of
the City.

After this the rebels assaulted the Palace of Herod, where many
had put their goods for safety, and driving out thence the Romans,
slew the people therein, and spoiled the place. Also they took two
soldiers, a horseman and a foot- soldier. The foot-soldier they slew
forthwith and dragged his body about the City, as if they would
avenge themselves upon him for all that the Romans had done to

them. As for the horseman, they bound his hands behind his back, and covered his eyes with a band, and made ready to slay him before the eyes of the Romans. But while the executioner was drawing his sword, the man escaped to the Romans. And Titus, because he had escaped from the enemy, would not slay him; but because he was not fit to be a soldier of Rome who had suffered himself to be taken alive, he commanded that they should strip him of his arms, and drive him out of the host.

The leaders of the rebels were the more obstinate in holding out, because they hoped that they should escape by hiding themselves in certain caverns that were under the earth. For they expected that search would not be made for them there; but that the Romans, when they had made an end of destroying the City, would depart, and they themselves could come forth. But this was a vain thought of theirs, that they should escape the vengeance of God and of their enemies. Nevertheless, because they had this hope, they increased daily in violence and cruelty.

After this, Titus began to set up banks for the taking of the Upper City. There was a great lack of timber for the works, for all the trees for the distance of a hundred furlongs from Jerusalem had been cut down for the former banks. Nevertheless the thing was done, the four legions building on the west side of the City, over against the Palace of Herod, and the auxiliaries and the mixed multitude building over against the Terrace and the bridge that was between the Upper City and the Temple, and the Tower of Sirnon, which he had built for a stronghold when he was fighting against John of Gischala.

In these days the captains of the Idumæans, assembling themselves in secret, took counsel whether they should not deliver themselves tip to Titus; and they sent five ambassadors to him, who should entreat him to have compassion upon them. And Titus, because he hoped that the rebels, when the Idumæans should have left them, who were their chief strength, would be willing to give themselves up, promised that he would give them their lives. But as they were preparing to depart, Simon perceived their purpose, and cast the captains into prison, having first slain the five men that had gone as

ambassadors to Titus. As for the common folk, he commanded that
they should be watched, and that the wall should be more diligently
kept, lest they should escape. Notwithstanding, though many were
slain, yet the greater part escaped. On these Titus had mercy and
saved their lives. The soldiers also were by this time wearied of slaying, and were willing to spare such as came to them, in the hope
of gain.

In these days a certain priest, named Joshua, when Titus had
sworn to him that he would save him alive, came forth and delivered
to him two candlesticks from the wall of the Temple, like to them that
were in the Holy Place, and tables also, and books, and cups; all of
which things were of gold throughout, and of a very great weight. He
also delivered to him curtains and garments of the priests, with
precious stones, and many other things that had been made for
ministering in the Temple. Moreover, the keeper of the treasury, by
name Phinehas, having been taken, showed where there lay tunics
and girdles of the priests, and a great store of purple dye and of
scarlet that was kept for the dyeing of the curtains, and also a very
great abundance of cinnamon and cassia and other spices, which
they were accustomed to mingle together for the making of the
incense that they offered in the Temple. Many other precious things
and ornaments of the Holy Place were delivered up by him, for the
sake of which things, though he had been taken by force, he received
mercy as if he had yielded himself.

On the seventh day of the month September, the siege-works
being now altogether finished (and this work was done in the space
of eighteen days), the Romans brought their machines near to the
Upper City. And when the rebels saw them, the most part being now
driven to despair, fled from the walls, and some hid themselves in the
caverns. Nevertheless there yet remained some who fought against
the men that had charge of the battering rams; but these were but few
in number and faint-hearted. And when a part of the wall had been
broken down, and some of the towers also had yielded to the
battering rams, these also fled. And now the leaders were in great
fear, for they saw no hope remaining to them. And first they sought to

break through the guards and so escape, but could not. And, indeed, it was as if God had turned their minds to folly by reason of their wickedness, for whereas, had they abode in the towers, they could never have been taken, save only from stress of hunger, they left these of their own accord, and hid themselves in the caverns.

Then did the Romans set up their standards upon the walls and celebrate their victory with great shouting and joy, having found the war, they said, easier at its ending than at its beginning. For this last wall of the City they took without any loss whatsoever, a thing almost beyond belief. Then they searched through the lanes and streets of the City, slaying all whom they met; and they burnt with fire many houses, with such as were therein. And in many of the houses, when they had gone into them seeking for plunder, they found whole families dead of hunger, and came forth from them with their hands empty. Nevertheless, though they felt some pity for the dead, they had no compassion upon the living, but slew them without mercy, till the streets were piled up with dead bodies. This they did until night-fall; and during the night the flames prevailed against the City, so that it was consumed altogether. And this befell on the eighteenth of the month September.

The next day Titus came into the City, and beheld it, marvelling much at the strength of the towers which the rebels had left of their own accord. And when he considered with himself how high they were, and how solidly built, and of how great stones, he said, "Surely now hath God been on our side, else the Jews had not left these towers; for, indeed, what could the hands of man do against them?" And when he commanded that the rest of the City should be destroyed, he would have these towers left, that they might be a memorial of his good fortune to them that should come after.

And now the soldiers being weary with slaying, seeing that a great multitude of the people yet remained alive, Titus commanded that they only should be put to death who had been found with arms upon them, and that the rest should be kept alive. But the soldiers slew, together with them whom they had been bidden to slay, the old men also and the weak. But such as were strong and in the vigour of their age they gathered together in the Court of the Women. Titus set one of his freedmen, Fronto by name, to have the charge of these, and to deal with them according to their deserts. Then Fronto commanded that all the rebels should be slain; yet he kept certain of the young men who surpassed the rest for beauty and stature against the triumph of Cæsar. Of them that remained he sent all that were of seventeen years and upwards to work in the mines of Egypt; but many were sent into the provinces to be slain by the sword and by wild beasts in the theatre. All such as were younger than seventeen years were sold. But a great multitude perished of hunger during these days, some because the guards for hatred would not give them to eat, and some because they would take nothing of their hands. And indeed there was not a sufficiency of food for so great a multitude.

Now the number of them that were taken captive was ninety-and-seven thousand in all; and the number of them that perished in the war was eleven-hundred- thousand. For a great multitude had assembled, according to custom, at the Feast of the Passover, and being overtaken suddenly by the war were not able to depart. And indeed, that so great a multitude could be gathered together in the City is manifest from the counting that was made in the days of Cestius. For when Nero made little account of the strength of the people, Cestius would have the priests take the number of the people. And they, when the Feast of the Passover was come, counted the number of the lambs that were slain for sacrifice; and the number was two-hundred-and-fifty-and-six thousand and five hundred; and for each lamb might be reckoned a company of ten men at the least. Nor are there counted herein such as were unclean, or the strangers that had come to the City for the Feast.

As for the leader of the rebels, John, being compelled by hunger, gave himself up to the Romans, and was saved alive, but kept in prison until the day of his death, but Simon they found not till after certain days. For when the Romans had taken the Upper City, this Simon, having with him certain of his friends whom he judged to be most faithful to himself, and with them stone-cutters, and tools such as were suitable for digging, and a great store of provisions, escaped into a cavern. And coming to the end of the cavern, he and his companions dug away the earth, for they hoped that when they had so dug for a certain space they might come forth into some safe place and so escape. But after making trial of the work they found that they had no hope of success. For the men that dug away the earth could do but little, and their food was well- nigh spent. Then Simon, seeking to astonish the Romans, and so escape them, put on him a white tunic and above it a purple robe, and came forth from the earth in the place where the Temple had stood. And at the first they that saw him stood still for wonder; but afterwards they went to him, and asked him who he was. This indeed he would not tell them, but bade them fetch their captain. Then they ran and fetched Terentius Rufus, for he had been left to command such part of the army as remained, for with the greater part Titus had already departed. Then Simon told the whole truth to Terentius, and Terentius kept him till he should hear the pleasure of Titus. The end of this Simon was that he was led as chief among the prisoners when Vespasian and Titus went in triumph to the Capitol in Rome, and that after the triumph he was slain.

Titus commanded that the whole City should be laid even with the ground, saving the three towers that were highest, even Phasælis, and Hippicos, and Mariamne, and a part of the wall that compassed the City towards the west; and these he left that they might show to the generations to come how great a city the Romans had taken.

After this he called together the whole army and made an oration to the soldiers, wherein he praised them greatly for their steadfastness and valour, declaring that not one who had borne himself bravely in the siege should go without his reward. Then he called to him such as had done any notable deeds of valour, and set crowns of gold upon their heads, and gave them also chains of gold, and long spears with shafts of gold, and ensigns of silver; and each man he promoted in his legion, or cohort, or squadron. After this he held a great sacrifice, wherein was slain a great multitude of oxen; and their flesh he gave to the soldiers for a feast. And after he had feasted with them for three days, he sent away the other legions, each to its proper place, but gave the charge of Jerusalem to the tenth.

After this he kept the birthday of his brother in the city of Cæsarea; and, as is the custom of the Romans at such feasts, he caused a great multitude of the Jews to be slain, constraining them to fight with each other, or with wild beasts. And not many days after he kept the birthday of his father in like manner. And this he did in the city of Berytus.

By this time Vespasian was come to Rome, and had been received as Emperor with good-will by the whole world; and he would that Titus should come to him without further delay. From Berytus therefore Titus went to Antioch, and from Antioch to Alexandria in Egypt. And as he was on his way to Alexandria he passed by the place where Jerusalem had been, and he was moved with compassion when he saw its desolation, that had been before more magnificent than all the cities of the world. At Alexandria he took ship and sailed into Italy, whither he had sent beforehand Simon and John, and others of the captives, to the number of seven hundred, being the tallest and fairest that could be found. When he was come near to Rome, his father Vespasian, having with him his younger son Domitian and a great multitude of the citizens, both small and great, came forth to meet him and conduct him into the city.

Not many days after, these two, even Vespasian and Titus, went, after the manner of the Romans, in a triumph to the Capitol. Now the manner of the triumph was this. While it was yet night all the soldiers that were in the city, being ranged in their squadrons and companies, surrounded the Temple of Isis; for there the Emperor and his son passed the night. And so soon as it was light the two came forth, having crowns of laurel about their heads, and clad in robes of purple after the manner of their country, and came to the terraces of Octavia, where the senate and the magistrates, and as many of the citizens as were of the rank of Knight, were assembled to meet them., There had been set a tribunal before the cloister, and on the tribunal two ivory chairs. On these they sat, being without armour or weapons, and the soldiers shouted when they saw them. After a while Vespasian beckoned with his hand that the shouting should be stayed; and there being made a great silence, he offered up prayer, according to custom, Titus also doing the same. And when he had made an end of praying, he bade the soldiers depart to the banquet which had been prepared for them; and he himself with Titus went without the city to the Gate of the Triumphs, which has its name because all triumphs pass through it. There, when they had taken some food, they were clad in robes of triumph, and after sacrifice done to the gods before the Gate, so passed into the city. And that the triumph might be the more easily seen of all the people. it was led through the theatres.

But to tell worthily the glory and splendour of that sight is not within the power of speech. For of all the riches that have ever been possessed of man there was nothing wanting that day to show the greatness of the Empire of Rome. Then might one see silver and gold and ivory in such plenty, that it seemed not as if some were carried for a show, but that all that there was in the whole world was gathered together in that one place. Also there was a great store of robes, of purple some of them, and some woven most skilfully in pictures; and jewels, set some in crowns of gold, and some in other works, and of all so many that one could no longer think them to be rare. There were carried also statues of the gods, of marvellous greatness and beauty, and not one of them that was not made of some precious stuff. After these came all kinds of animals, each adorned after his kind. And the men that carried these things had purple robes and crowns of gold. Also there were to be seen the prisoners that had been kept for the triumph, all very splendidly adorned, and the splendour and variety of their equipment was such that men noted not their weariness and misery. Nor was there anything more marvellous than the greatness and height of the carriages on which all these things were borne, being some of them of three or even four stories. And on the sides of the carriages there were pictures of all kinds of warfare, marvellously well wrought. There could men see the laying waste of some fertile country, and the slaying of great hosts of the enemy; for some could be seen to flee, and some to be led into captivity; and great walls were broken down by machines, and cities full of inhabitants taken by force, and armies entered in, with other such like sights. And on each carriage was the chief of the city that had been taken.

Of all the spoils of war that were borne in the triumph, the richest and most beautiful were they that had been taken from the Temple at Jerusalem, among which was a table of gold of many talents in weight, and a candle-stick of gold, having seven branches, according to the number which the Jews are wont to have in the highest honour; and after the candlestick the Book of the Law. After all the spoils came the Emperor Vespasian, and next to Vespasian was Titus his son. With these also went Domitian; and in this array they came to the Temple of Jupiter of the Capitol.

After this Vespasian built a Temple of Peace; and in this he laid up the vessels that had been taken from the Temple; but the veil of the Temple and the Book of the Law were laid up in the Palace.